MEDICAL PRACTICE MANAGEMENT DESK BOOK

Charles H. Walsh, C.P.B.C.
and
Morton Walker, D.P.M.

PRENTICE-HALL, INC.
ENGLEWOOD CLIFFS, NEW JERSEY

Prentice-Hall International, Inc., *London*
Prentice-Hall of Australia, Pty. Ltd., *Sydney*
Prentice-Hall of Canada, Ltd., *Toronto*
Prentice-Hall of India Private Ltd., *New Delhi*
Prentice-Hall of Japan, Inc., *Tokyo*
Prentice-Hall of Southeast Asia Pte. Ltd., *Singapore*
Whitehall Books, Ltd., *Wellington, New Zealand*

© 1982 by
Prentice-Hall, Inc.
Englewood Cliffs, N.J.

All rights reserved. No part of this book may be reproduced in any form or by any means without permission in writing from the publisher.

Library of Congress Cataloging in Publication Data

Walsh, Charles H.
  Medical practice management desk book.

  Includes bibliographical references and index.
  1. Medicine—Practice. I. Walker, Morton. II. Title.
R728.W34   610'.68   81-19972
                           AACR2

ISBN 0-13-572701-4

Printed in the United States of America

GERALD E. SWANSON, M.D.
9601 UPTON ROAD
MINNEAPOLIS, MN 55431
TELE: 881-6869

To Sophia, Charlie, and Julia, for their encouragement, enthusiasm, motivation, understanding, and contagious spirit of achievement

and

Melvin J. Goldberg, who has faithfully propagated the principles of medical practice management.

About the Authors

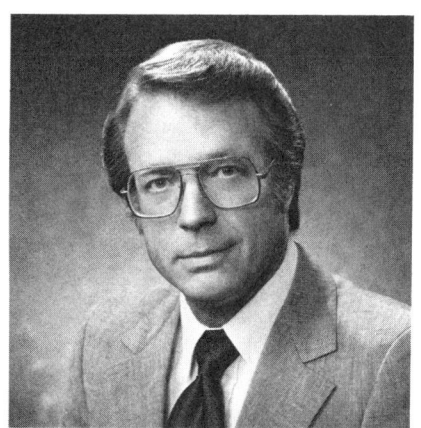

Charles H. Walsh, C.P.B.C. is the founder and president of the management consulting firm, Associated Professional Consultants, Inc., Elmhurst, Illinois, which serves more than four hundred doctors. He is a Certified Professional Business Consultant with twenty years experience as a physician's consultant and is a former president of the National Society of Medical-Dental Management Consultants. He is Chairman of the Board of Governors of Memorial Hospital of DuPage County, Illinois.

A graduate of Northwestern University, with several years' post-graduate work to his credit, Mr. Walsh resides in Elmhurst, Illinois with his wife, Sophia, and two children, Charles and Julia. He is an active member of his community serving on several church, school and local executive committees. He has lectured at Loyola University School of Medicine, the Illinois College of Podiatric Medicine, and the Illinois Institute for Continuing Legal Education. He recently completed a lecture tour for Seminars and Symposia.

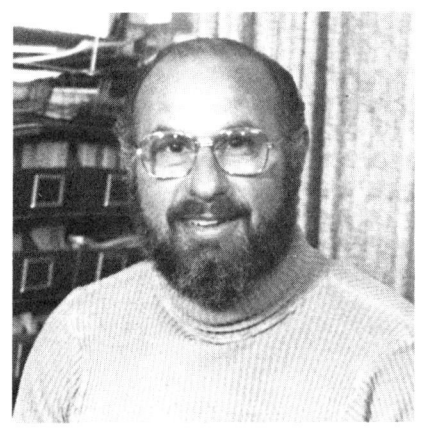

Dr. Morton Walker is a professional freelance medical journalist who left the practice of podiatric medicine thirteen years ago. He is the author of seventeen published books on health subjects and some thousand magazine articles. He has done medical ghostwriting for doctors in many fields and is published in *Drug Therapy Medical Journal, Dental Management, Optometric Management, Physician's Management, Practical Psychology for Physicians, the Journal of the American Podiatry Association*, and other journals.

Dr. Walker is the recipient of twenty-one medical writing and business writing awards, among them two Jesse H. Neal Editorial Achievement Awards from the American Business Press, Inc. One was for writing the best series of magazine articles published in 1975; the second was for writing and editing the best special magazine issue published in 1976. In 1979, the American Academy of Medical Preventics presented him with "The Humanitarian Award" "for informing the American public on alternative methods of healing." The Institute of Preventive Medicine, Washington, D.C., made Dr. Walker the recipient of the "Orthomolecular Award" of 1981 "for outstanding achievement in orthomolecular education. In the face of adversity you have persevered giving new meaning to the right of each citizen to choose his own medical treatment." He has won the American Podiatry Association's highest award, its fiftieth anniversary gold medal for research and writing.

Dr. Walker works at home in Stamford, Connecticut. His son, Mark, is a fifth year resident in general surgery. His son, Randall, is a certified public accountant for a "Fortune 500" corporation. His son, Jules, is a senior in high school. Dr. Walker is married to Joan for thirty-two years, and she is a radio commentator and lecturer.

How This Desk Book Can Boost Your Medical Practice Income And Personal Payoff

Offshore of the Cayman Islands, most westerly in the blue Caribbean, barrel-chested skin divers search crystalline waters for living conch shells. Time after time they bring up armloads of mollusks in hopes that one might contain a pearl to fetch a price. There is no way to tell in advance which conch bears a pearly nugget. Divers may plunge for days at a time and acquire only edible mollusk meat for making chowder and stew to sustain hungry families. Only the law of averages dictates an occasional uncovering of a pearl within fleshy mollusk folds. The more pink conch shells they bring to the surface, the more pearls they are likely to find.

Managing a successful medical practice today faces a course parallel to diving for conch among the Caymanians. Your family security and financial rewards are predicated in part upon repeated diving into unknown depths. Your conch shells are your patients. Your family's edible mollusk meats are represented by the services you dispense. But the pearls! Ah, the pearls are the investment returns from your studious financial investigation, your sound management judgment, your wise economic decisions.

Do you ascend from the depths carrying armloads of pearl-bearing conch?

This *Medical Practice Management Desk Book* is your manned small submersible to help you reap submerged riches. It provides the information foundation with which to erect your skyscraper to prosperity. Within this handy, easy-to-use volume, you will uncover current and practical solutions to most practice management problems.

The coauthors have supplied new, original, and innovative information. Various systems, short cuts, checklists, facts, ideas, unique methods, time-saving procedures, forms, tables, illustrations, and much more show you how to boost your practice income without sacrificing professional standards of excellence. Chapters in this desk book offer case histories taken from the daily practice lives of health care professionals. (To respect the privacy of the individuals involved in some of these case examples, names have been slightly changed.)

The dynamic money acquisition tips packed into forthcoming chapters, in fact, come mostly from expertise derived from the management of over 1,000 clients practicing in successful health care offices. Tested and proven management techniques are contributed by many professional practice consultants and doctors, themselves. With the ownership of this desk reference book, you will immediately possess instant retrieval in detail of the best office controls, maximum personnel productivity, higher gross income, lower materials waste, and greater profits from practice and professional corporate growth.

37 REASONS WHY THIS BOOK WILL HELP YOU MANAGE MORE PROFITABLY

The *Medical Practice Management Desk Book* is crammed full of special income-producing, clear-cut, rock solid practice management steps, procedures, systems techniques, examples, and checklists. Here are just a few of the valuable items contained in this text.

- How to determine if a community will support a profitable practice.
- 12 strategic management approaches to developing a practice.
- 14 daily audits your business manager should make.
- What you should expect from a practice management consultant.
- 30 benefits from constructive patient feedback.
- 7 basic personality traits for a humanized practice.
- 10 commandments of human relations.
- 10 ethical principals for making major money.
- Pondering 13 questions that help capture referrals.
- Learn the characteristics of the suit-prone patient to avoid becoming a suit-prone doctor.
- 10-point checklist to prevent malpractice claims.
- Are you a groupie or too rugged an individualist to flex in a professional joint venture—Chapter 5 gives pros and cons.
- What are the secrets of successful partners.
- 6 group practice benefits for patients.
- 10 advantages of group practice and 10 disadvantages.
- Be the "good doctor" and answer the 5 basic questions every patient wants answered.
- At what point should you consider a corporate structure for your practice.
- The 7 most common questions asked about medical incorporation.
- 15 recommended changes in office procedure and management of a professional service corporation.
- 23 items to help you compare business structures and retirement plans.
- How do office patterns work—21 considerations.
- 32 tips for saving your time.
- 7 hints for utilizing the office staff's time when you are away, with 10 tasks to be accomplished.
- Personnel policies that work.
- Tips on interviewing potential employees.
- Delegating responsibilities will enable you to attain that $250,000 net.

- A no-waste inventory control system that's simple and quick.
- 3 steps to stating your fees without feeling guilt.
- Capital capacity, character, conditions = credit.
- 9 danger signals of deadbeats.
- The 5-month follow-up billing procedure.
- 6 effective sample collection letters for follow-up of delinquent accounts.
- 8 guidelines in selecting a collection agency.
- How much should you earn?
- If "budget" sounds too confining, try "planned expenditure programming."
- Maxwell Maltz's acronym of S U C C E S S.
- Get involved with your financial goals.

MORE BIG DOLLAR SAVINGS IN CASH AND TIME

The Art of Professional Practice Management reduces the toll on your mind and body taken by poorly administered human relations. Combining the methods of business with the ethics of professionalism is an art. Proper application of this art saves you several absolutely nonexpendable practice components—namely, your heart, your psyche, your time. For doctor-saving support look within these pages (Chapter 1).

Collections must be included in any talk about big dollar losses. There was a time when a man's word was enough to bind an agreement—you rendered service, you got paid—but, no more. To be compensated for your professional skill, years of schooling, investment in facilities and equipment, collection management must now come into play (Chapters 7 and 9).

If you are currently caught in a squeeze between higher operating costs and limited fee-for-service increases, must borrow money to operate or expand, feel like you're a kind of financial agency for certain patients, read what's written here. We will help solve problems of office expense, fee structure, low earnings, mixed up financial records, and overdue accounts receivable.

Malpractice suits with their skyrocketing awards and the high-priced professional liability insurance premiums to protect you against them, give you swift kicks in the wallet. All signs indicate that unless some radical changes in laws or procedures take place, whopping awards, a greater number of claims, and constant rate hikes in malpractice coverage are going to be annual events (Chapter 4).

Have you wondered if there's a fair way out? Are you seriously considering giving up solo practice for the built-in peer review protection of a group? Do you worry about how to keep disgruntled patients from suing? Maybe for the sheer security of practicing that way, an H.M.O. is in your future. The conflict is wearing. Many solutions will be found in this book (Chapter 5).

Consultation—the master's discipline—a way to keep more of what you make and make more of what you keep without working harder. Frequently, working harder is next to impossible for the average doctor, anyway. But consulting makes practice life a pleasure, and this book tells you how to go about building a consulting practice or how to apply consultant talent to ease the burdens of patient care (Chapter 3).

Accounting for the doctor can hold much creative satisfaction, especially when you're counting practice profits. In this *Medical Practice Management Desk Book,* financial subjects that might have been dry are "served up juicy." For example, we show you how to supply information on demand to government agencies, bankers, creditors, investors, and other outside interests. In a flash you know costs of current office operation without any entries askew. In turn, you will learn how to understand the growth patterns of an enterprise you may wish to invest in.

Enjoy accounting at last with properly organized systems backed by suitable records. Own a layout of methods and procedures to implement the systems. Teach yourself accounting to interpret results. In a conversational format, we demonstrate how to accomplish business transaction analysis and professional practice recording (Chapter 7).

Health care cost-cutting within the next few years will blast your combination lock right off the wall safe door. Consumer advocates and the Federal government are looking at differences in aggregate fees and payments to family physicians versus internists; pediatricians against pathologists; psychiatrists as opposed to neurologists; general surgeons versus vascular surgeons, etc. They want to be shown justification for the giant differences in payments to specialists and general physicians.

No wonder you face the glut of health insurance forms and other paperwork. Medicare and "Fedicare" are already controlling your fees. To be decided next is what income you should be allowed to make. Are you going to let this happen?

WHO HANDLES YOUR PRACTICE MANAGEMENT?

Advances in medical science and technology—computerized histories, multiphasic screening, hospital based facilities, scientific diagnosis and treatment—have you practicing quality modern medicine. It's what you were trained to do. But all your science and art of medicine can die from poorly administered professional practice management.

Who handles your practice management, doctor? Do you pass problems of plugging financial leaks, the planning of insurance protection, the borrowing of money, the art of human relations in collection management, and the other principles of practice management to one of your office workers?

If you could have a choice—full and final success or the ongoing struggle to climb rungs to the top of the professional ladder—which would you want? You would probably choose the problem of success; but you *might* be making a mistake.

Why? Because the conduct that won your full and final achievement is often abandoned when you attain the top. It becomes usual for you to accept less efficient methods. It's a time when you let down on the best methods of medical practice management.

Aside from the doctor with an "average" practice, the physician at his pinnacle will find this desk book useful. We have organized our book into 12 practice-boosting chapters. Each one is structured to help you reach an unreached goal.

The great lyric poet Horace put it this way: "Adversity has the effect of eliciting talents which in prosperous circumstances would have lain dormant."

That's why we have written a financial reference book that won't let your motivation become vacillating. Success can slow you down. But poor practice management can wear you out and waste you to death. When you lift this book from your desk and read it for reference, you'll become infused with renewed motivation. The book has you sidestep pitfalls and avoid all manner of mistakes in matters of money. Using the information between its covers makes a poor practice good and a good practice ideal.

Like the skin divers of the Cayman Islands who explore for conch in the warm, blue sea, your own search for knowledge in these pages must eventually net you pearls of wisdom. At least, be assured that, just like the Caymanian family men, you will always come up with good edible meat.

Now dive right in and retrieve the income-adding, estate-building, practice-boosting pearls you seek. The chapters that follow are worthy of your time—and your money.

(Please note: text references are listed at the end of each chapter where they occur.)

Charles H. Walsh, C.P.B.C.
Morton Walker, D.P.M.

Contents

How This Desk Book Can Boost Your Medical Practice Income
And Personal Payoff   9

chapter one

Grossing a Quarter-Million-a-Year and More in Medical Practice   19

    Figuring the Feasability of $250,000 a Year – 22
    Twelve Strategic Management Approaches – 22
    The Medical Practice Audit – 28
    Do You Need a Business Manager? – 29
    How to Get Your Money's Worth from a Practice
    Consultant – 32

chapter two

Humanizing Patient Care Brings Big Dollar Earnings   35

    How to Overcome Imperception and Get Patient
    Feedback – 39
    Thirty Benefits from Constructive Patient
    Feedback – 39
    Seven Basic Personality Traits for a Humanized
    Practice – 42
    The Ten Commandments of Human Relations – 43
    References for Chapter Two – 46

chapter three

Applying Secrets of Salesmanship Multiplies Patient Referrals   47

    Friendly Competition in Medical Practice – 49
    Ten Ethical Principles for Making Major Money – 50

How to Gain Acceptance by the Medical
Community – 51
Patient Referrals from Certain Actions – 52
The Effect of Attitude on Practice Growth – 55
Thirteen Questions to Ask About Your
Referrals – 56
Is Your Practice Run Like a Chinese Laundry? – 57
The ABCs for Stimulating More Referrals from
Key Patients – 57

chapter four

17 Ways to Shield Doctors from Devastating Malpractice Suits — 59

One of the First U.S. Medical Malpractice
Decisions – 61
How Special Interest Groups See It – 62
Every Fourth Physician Is Hit by Malpractice
Claims – 62
Why Patients Sue Their Physicians – 64
Are You a Suit-Prone Doctor? – 64
Characteristics of the Suit-Prone Patient – 65
Guidelines for Evaluation of the Anxiety-Ridden
Patient – 66
The Real Reason Patients Sue Doctors – 68
The Ten-Point Patient Checklist to Prevent
Malpractice Claims – 69
The Menace of Practicing Defensive Medicine – 70
Preventing Excessive Court Awards with the
Medical Malpractice Accident Fund – 72
References for Chapter Four – 73

chapter five

Picking the Medical Practice Formation That Reaps A Quarter-Million-a-Year — 75

Motivators for Joining Corporate Medicine – 78
Might You Be a Solo Country Doctor? – 78
Joint Ventures in Medical Practice – 83
Joining a Medical Group – 86
Reference for Chapter Five – 91

CONTENTS

chapter six

Net More of Your $250,000 Annual Gross This Doctor-Proven Way — 93

    Why Consider Incorporating at All? – 95
    The Establishment of ERISA – 96
    There Are Many Advantages of an Incorporated Practice – 96
    What Does Formation of a Professional Corporation Cost? – 99
    Recommended Changes in Office Procedure and Management for Your New Professional Service Corporation – 100
    Self-Employed (Keogh) Plans – 102
    The Corporate Retirement Program Compared to a Keogh Program – 102

chapter seven

55 Medical Practice Management Action Ideas with High Six-Figure Potential — 109

    The Four "Ps" of Ideal Medical Practice Management – 111
    The First "P" of Practice Management: Your Patient – 112
    The Second "P" of Practice Management: You, the Physician – 115
    The Third "P" of Practice Management: Supporting Personnel – 120
    The Fourth "P" of Practice Management: Office Procedures – 133
    Reference for Chapter Seven – 136

chapter eight

Galvanizing Employees to Accelerate Income — 137

    Delegating by the Clinical Task Checklist – 140
    A Checklist of Office Tasks Which Can Be Delegated – 142
    Having an Inventory System That Allows No Waste – 144

Do You Have All the Equipment You Need? – 147
Avoiding Nonproductive Office Time – 147

chapter nine

What Every Profit-Minded Doctor Should Know About Setting Fees and Collecting Bills 149

Charging the Fairest Way – 152
Do Your Services Cost Too Much? – 153
How to Present Your Fee – 154
The Ongoing Battle Over Fees – 155
Changing Times for Health Care Credit – 156
Your Office Policy in Business Matters – 156
The Four "Cs" of a Patient Credit Application – 157
How to Use Your Community Credit Bureau – 158
Nine Danger Signals of Deadbeats – 159
The Best Collection Procedure for Slow-Paying Patients – 160
Samples of Effective Collection Letters – 162
How to Follow Up Delinquent Accounts – 163
Eight Guidelines in Selecting a Collection Agency – 164
Should You Try to Collect by Legal Action? – 165
Receiving Up-Front Funding By Factoring – 166
References for Chapter Nine – 166

chapter ten

Skyrocket Medical Practice Net Income by Budgeting Office Expense 167

How Much Should You—or Anyone Else—Earn? – 170
Do You Keep the Fullest Percentage After You Earn It? – 171
Why You May Not Keep Much of What You Earn – 172
The Bright Future for Incorporated Professionals – 173
Practice Philosophy Determines Your Life Style – 173
Let a Bank Automate Your Financial Records – 174

CONTENTS

The Payoff of Expense Sharing – 175
Adopting the Success Philosophy of Maxwell Maltz – 176
References for Chapter Ten – 177

chapter eleven

How to Get Your Personal Finances in Step with This Six-Figure Target   179

Interpretation of the Personal Statement – 181
Estate Planning – 185
Necessary Steps in Estate Planning 185
Creating an Estate Trust – 187

chapter twelve

How Corporate Pension Plans Help You Reach the Quarter-Million Goal   189

Index   199

chapter one

Grossing
A Quarter-Million-a-Year and More
In Medical Practice

Our greatest asset is our dignity and self respect. We keep saying that this is the land of opportunity. But we must stop teaching that opportunity knocks. It never knocks. You can listen at the door for ten lifetimes, but you won't hear it knocking. You are opportunity. You open the door.

— Maxwell Maltz, M.D., 1968

What's your financial goal? Is your practice bringing in $250,000 a year without your struggling against time and patient relations problems? A quarter million dollars annually is being grossed in other offices throughout the country by individual doctors of character who have competence not only in professional skill but also in practice management.

What is practice management? It isn't only getting work done efficiently by using employees, systems, manipulations, simplistic approaches, and authoritarianism. Rather, it is the purposive application of the techniques of planning, organizing, integrating, measuring, and setting goals for your business effort.

Managing your medical practice can have you grossing a quarter of a million dollars yearly.

Case in Point: Soon after Medicare came in, most members of the American College of Radiology went about securing different financial agreements with hospitals than was usual until then. The typical arrangement in 1966 was a 35 percent payment from the hospital of the radiological department's total production. The hospitals were frankly enjoying the relationship and making more money by somewhat subordinating these specialists.

Two radiologists in partnership, Morgan Flintner and Adam Saxton of Providence, Rhode Island, instituted management practices to increase their annual gross incomes. They were each bringing in approximately $40,000.

Flintner and Saxton presented their case for separate billing to the board of trustees of the hospital in order to establish a fee for service for the various radiological procedures. Using the old-time relative value scale, they developed a fee schedule and, with the hospital's concurrence, established a separate in-house controlled billing system. Thus, the radiologists set up their own business and in less than two years doubled their income. Now, fifteen years later, they are splitting a gross annual income of one-half million dollars.

FIGURING THE FEASIBILITY OF $250,000 A YEAR

Figure your financial goal feasibility by adapting the same technique used by real estate business people and stock analysts. They often refer to the "P/E Ratio" when they evaluate a piece of property. "P" stands for "Price"; "E" designates "Earnings." You may adapt this P/E ratio to mean your "Physician's/Earnings Ratio."

Management consultants generally agree that the specialist in family practice can accommodate a patient population of 2,000. On the other hand, it takes at least 7,000 people to support a solo internist, obstetrician/gynecologist, one general surgeon, or a single pediatrician. Other specialists who are not hospital-based require a patient population per physician of about 15,000.

Just as do real estate investors, you must look at the community to decide if it will support a profitable practice by its having a high P/E ratio.

Here are some of the questions you should answer in making a P/E evaluation:

- Is the population attuned to your kind of practice?
- Does the community offer employment to people in many diversified fields?
- Are there any ethnic barriers between you and your general run of patients?
- Does the community exhibit solid, permanent growth with evidence of people buying homes?
- Are Medicaid and Medicare disbursements made efficiently and without hassle?
- Does the area provide a lifestyle—urban, suburban, rural—of the type you will be happy with?
- Are personal income statistics of residents indicative of their ability to pay for your services?
- Does the volume of local retail show a community in good economic health?

Typical P/E ratio questions such as these need answers before you can determine the feasibility of earning $250,000 a year in the particular city, town or village where you plan to expand an existing practice or where you desire to settle initially. Having affirmed the feasibility of an area's growth, the next step is to examine your practice carefully.

TWELVE STRATEGIC MANAGEMENT APPROACHES

It may be a cliché to mention that the need for technical competence is ever-increasing in modern medical practice. Yet, some physicians are willing to provide superb professional service without considering the management aspects of the private practice of medicine. Their attitude is "Let the office assistants take care of practice management—I'll stick to medicine because that's what I'm trained to do."

This is a book about individual practice management that will earn you upwards of $250,000 annually. As a physician you have a professional obligation to make your skills available to as many people as possible and bring you fulfillment of your goals. You can do this by instituting the *S.M.A.-12,* which refers to the twelve *Strategic Management Approaches of excellent practice management.* They will help you develop your practice according to your own personality, skills, and interests.

The S.M.A.-12 will assure your building a practice with steady and gradual growth. It will come as no surprise when you increase your patient load, expand office facilities, and realize your full potential for providing the best medical service you have at your command. Then you will feel inner satisfaction that you are fulfilling your destiny. If you cannot do this, if you constantly find yourself beset by organizational and financial difficulties, you won't be able to provide the medical care you have been trained to deliver. In effect, better medical practice management means better medical care for your patients.

S.M.A. Number One – Location

The location of your office is the single most important evaluation you can make relating to the character of your practice. You will have asked yourself if there is a need and acceptance of your type of practice in the community. Here are thirteen other specific questions to answer concerning practice location.

1. Are other professional offices in my local area creating a sort of "doctor's row" or is my practice in a professional office building?
2. Do current zoning laws tend to protect the neighborhood and my investment in the location?
3. Are the long-established people in the neighborhood tending to stay put?
4. Does the neighborhood show signs of upgrading with new buildings and stores or new homes?
5. Is the location of my practice near my home without an annoying or time-consuming commute?
6. Is the traffic flow efficiently dispersed by suitable road width and traffic aids?
7. Is my office street a main artery known to almost everyone in the community?
8. Is there public transportation nearby?
9. Do I have adequate parking for patients who come by car?
10. Is there adequacy of office space or the opportunity for expansion should my practice grow?

11. Are there sufficient skilled personnel available and ready to be employed if I should need them?
12. Are accessory facilities such as pharmacies, hospitals, ambulance services and other professional consultants convenient to my location?
13. Is the quality of the space itself representative of the dignity of the medical profession? Will it attract the type of patient I would like to treat?

S.M.A. Number Two – Patient Relations

Your manner of handling people, rather than your medical acumen, is generally what will get you patient referrals, and that is where good patient relationships play a role.

If you answer "No" to any of the following ten questions, you need help and an honest analysis of your patient relations attitude:

1. Am I available by telephone at all times?
2. Do I think in terms of referrals?
3. Am I punctual in keeping appointments?
4. Are my appointments made for more than two weeks in advance?
5. Do I discuss fees with patients prior to performing services that would be out of the ordinary routine?
6. Are my fees at a matching scale with fees charged by others in the area for services similar to mine?
7. Do I discuss payment on delinquent accounts with patients?
8. Are discussions between the patient and my secretary held in private?
9. Do I permit or invite my patient to reveal his fear of fees or procedures?
10. Do I sympathize and reassure the patient that his reaction is an understandable one and then go on to calm the reaction?

S.M.A. Number Three – Office Design

The treatment facility itself should have the best possible layout provided by the space. Patients who visit your office for the first time may be impressed by what they see because of a prevailing atmosphere of progressive medicine being practiced. Without a doubt, people tend to form an opinion of your personality, your professional attitude, your outlook on life, and even your competence as a doctor by the kind of treatment facility that represents you.

Tips in Office Design:
• A physician generally needs approximately one thousand square feet to function effectively.
• The reception room should display a wise selection of color, comfortable seating, tasteful lighting, and have wall to wall carpeting or well-polished floors. The reception room should accommodate at least three times the number of people you see per hour. The patients must have easy access to the receptionist, and

the receptionist must have sight control of the entire reception area. Individual seating is preferable to couches, sofas or love seats. Make sure that chairs have arms. You need about ten square feet per seat. Background music is a pleasant added feature along with current magazines. Don't overlook supplying educational medical literature for this room.

• A good-sized examination room measures about 100 square feet altogether, probably ten feet by ten feet. Each examination room should be identical in layout, design and equipment. (The examination table may best be set diagonally in the room to allow for walking around it and having the patient's head closest to the entry door.) Place a chart rack outside each examination room and have some signaling device installed to indicate the status of that room at any given time.

Rule: Know where the staff and patients are at all times.

S.M.A. Number Four – Systems and Policies

Office systems and utilization start with a well-controlled accounting system, possibly a quite elaborate method. We will get to that kind of accounting system later in this book.

You should be able to answer affirmatively the following eleven questions:

1. Does my receptionist or assistant fill out a day sheet, a kind of diary of the day's office activity?
2. Does he or she keep an advance appointment book?
3. Do I have a good business filing system working?
4. Are there careful controls of accounts receivable?
5. Does my office have an effective delinquency policy?
6. Are my patients billed each month?
7. Does my staff issue written instructions to patients when indicated?
8. Do they screen my incoming telephone calls?
9. Is office utilization tied into my regular office hours?
10. Is my need to visit the hospital taken into consideration when patients are scheduled for office visits?
11. Is there an understanding with my staff members and patients as to what the patient is supposed to do in the event of an emergency?

S.M.A. Number Five – Furnishings and Equipment

Your equipment and furnishings should be kept current and up to the latest standards, not only in effectiveness but in style. Without question, it is in your power to make the practice of medicine more enjoyable for yourself by performing your professional function with first-rate equipment. There is no reason to practice with anything less than something approaching the ideal; you will reap the final benefits in the form of professional pride and self-confidence. This confidence will carry over to your patients and in their turn, they will refer other patients with confidence.

Additionally, a chair with a broken arm or a threadbare piece of carpet on the floor does not do anything to lift your status in the patient's eyes. Clean and up-to-date furnishings really do hold great import for how you feel about your office and how patients feel about you.

Some doctors tend to get accustomed to working with outmoded equipment and shoddy furnishings. They don't recognize some poorly styled pieces of apparatus and fail to see these items the way patients see them.

Note: Bring in an objective observer to give an opinion about what he or she thinks of your office's appearance.

> *Case in Point:* Robert A. Jordan, M.D., of Addison, Illinois did this prior to refurbishing his business and control areas. Dr. Jordan, an obstetrician/gynecologist, had what appeared to be a well-appointed office, but it lacked privacy for patients in the business areas. He sought the services of David J. Wellehan, a certified professional business management consultant, and received an opinion for making alterations that were focused on the needs of an ob./gyn. practice.
>
> Even though an architect had already laid out changes for the business area, Dr. Jordan scrapped these plans and went beyond them. Following Mr. Wellehan's advice, the design was reworked, walls were repartitioned, and other adjustments were made. The new layout brought benefits that the doctor hadn't imagined initially. His staff's business efficiency increased measurably. He saw the improvement in speed of patient flow and better collections. Patients no longer were reticent to talk about money matters and appointment schedules. The staff opened up, too.
>
> Dr. Jordan's experience is illustrative of the need to secure professional advice outside your area of expertise. In the same way that you seek consultation in medicine, you should seek it in financial transactions as well.

S.M.A. Number Six – Patient Perceptions

Public relations in practice involves building a professional image through communication. There are many forms of communication, of course. The most vital is that which is done personally with patients.

Each patient should understand exactly what you are saying. When you speak of diagnosis and prescribe treatment do you use language that is difficult to understand? Your reply should be a loud "no," because you talk plainly and descriptively.

In professional or social contacts, on the street, at the supermarket, in church, or at the theater, your patients and neighbors will expect of you that type of behavior and speech which is consistent with their perception of a physician. What is needed in this case is to recognize what perception they have and live up to it. Your role is to act and speak at the level of communication most acceptable and understandable to the individual you are confronting.

S.M.A. Number Seven – Professional Relations

Professional relations include not only contacts and consultations with other physicians but also hospital affiliations and emergency room use. Emergency rooms are practice builders. They afford you an especially good exposure for purposes of referral and practice growth, since they are places where other physicians can see you in action.

The best way to become known in the medical community is through association with as many medical groups compatible with your time and commitments.

If you find yourself faced with a choice of hospital affiliations, the deciding factor could be one of the following:

A. The facility identified with your religious group,

B. The one located nearer to you,

C. The hospital where you interned,

D. The one with the best facilities for your practice specialty.

S.M.A. Number Eight – Auxiliary Patient Care Facilities

You and the various local health agencies derive mutual benefits from co-operative efforts.

Familiarize yourself with the auxiliary health facilities in your community such as convalescent homes, The Visiting Nurse Association, home health aides and homemaker services, family and children's agencies, the Red Cross, and others. Actively participate in the outpatient and ward services of at least two local hospitals. Give some clinical teaching time on a voluntary basis in a hospital affiliated with a medical school.

Perhaps you could do volunteer work in a youth center, mental health center or other program. Cover for other physicians also. Certainly, any doctor who is interested in the growth of his practice should become acquainted with most of the physicians in his medical community.

S.M.A. Number Nine – Third Party Involvements

Insurance companies are a source of income through several means. As the third party involved in medical care, health insurance companies often make patient payments.

You can apply to one or more of them for an appointment to become an insurance medical examiner. Not only does such an appointment provide a source of income, but it also generates new patients. People have a tendency to continue with the insurance company doctor who has examined them and taken their health history, if they don't already have their own physician.

S.M.A. Number Ten – Say "Thank You"

Acknowledgments made to people who refer patients to you encourages these people to send you more patients. Elementary as this sounds, many professionals consider themselves too busy or their time too valuable to spend it thanking people. Certainly a major way to build referrals from colleagues is to send carefully written notes about each patient seen to the physician who has sent that patient.

Express gratitude in person or in writing also to your patients who refer others. Plant seeds of gratitude and they will sprout into a harvest of patients to nourish your practice.

S.M.A. Number Eleven – Perform Community Work

Community involvements should include not only the doctor but his or her spouse as well. A spouse is an important part of your practice plan—a helpmate to do some entertaining community work.

Various extra activities such as being available to lecture to local service groups or being the doctor on call at local school football games are community involvements that you can elect for yourself.

S.M.A. Number Twelve – Contract for Your Services

Medical service contracts can be quite lucrative and rewarding from the standpoint of building a practice. Dealings with industrial accounts or schools provide you with a fresh supply of patients simply because an individual is likely to stay with the doctor who performs a service for him when he does not have his own physician.

Having adopted these *twelve strategic management approaches to practice management,* you will have embarked upon a game plan by which your medical practice will thrive and grow. Each of the twelve guidelines adopted will better establish you as an effective practice manager and business entrepreneur. You'll surely reap the reward of a quarter of a million dollars or more of gross annual income.

Our *S.M.A.-12* will establish an achievement orientation in your office for creation of more long-range plans for practice growth. They are motivators—catalysts—that multiply all practice assets. Unless the definition of luck includes preparation to meet opportunity, very few accomplishments come about through luck. So, you will orient yourself and your staff to recognize opportunity when it comes knocking. As Maxwell Maltz said, "*You* are opportunity. *You* open the door."

THE MEDICAL PRACTICE AUDIT

Opening the door to opportunity comes with your not only being a doctor but also a practice administrator. This means you need to feel an enthusiastic sense of self-worth. You must be a businessperson, personnel director, patient educator, empathetic counselor, psychologist and an individual upholding the image of a professional. To assume all these roles is no easy matter. It calls for a personal daily checklist, something we call *the medical practice audit.* Accordingly we have prepared the following six questions which fulfill some self-imposed requirements of the practicing physician.

Ask yourself these questions at the end of every day:

1. Have I recognized and coped with personal traits of my patients and personnel?
2. Have I counteracted difficulties involving fees, payments, interpersonal communications, appointments, and other aspects of patient contact?
3. Have I satisfactorily eliminated any causes of patient complaints?
4. Have I explained administrative and fiscal policies to patients and/or staff?
5. Have I accomplished what I intended to do today and taken a step closer to my specific practice goals?
6. Have I done something nice for someone today, including myself?

DO YOU NEED A BUSINESS MANAGER?

There is no reason why you should take up office systems and procedures as a hobby. Making appointments, posting for bookkeeping, and marking account cards are tedious, low-paid tasks and a waste of your valuable time. You will be wise to delegate these jobs to someone else just as soon as the right individual shows up to do them. That individual is the medical practice business manager. He or she must be able to relieve you of administrative responsibilities and free you for greater earnings through rendering medical services.

Do you think you need a business manager to do the following: Take charge of patient appointment emergencies, manage collections, check credits, keep account books, write recalls and patient letters, adjust complaints, investigate new equipment, hire personnel, make sure of insurance protection, purchase supplies, pay bills, and generally run the office? Are you willing to dilute your patient appointment time to do all these various administrative jobs? No? Then you need a business manager!

> *Case in Point:* David Young, M.D. of Chicago, an internist, eventually recognized his need for help in managing the business affairs of his office. He knew that a business manager would be valuable, so he hired Mrs. Phyllis Bradshaw to fill the job. Dr. Young had been plagued with excessive personnel turnover. He was overloaded with expensive and cumbersome systems and procedures that were throwing his ratio of expenses to earnings out of kilter. The resulting disorganization finally became a serious situation.
>
> Mrs. Bradshaw, a firm individual with strength and depth in business management, came on board the seasick practice. She instituted simplified yet controlled systems to effect a smoothly run office. She wrote job descriptions for the internist's new employee manuals, and these altered the hiring procedures. The employees are now content.

Dr. Young currently finds himself free to devote primary time to his patients without the former hassles of office management. Still, he is more firmly in control than ever before and is earning beyond the $250,000 a year he wants for himself.

Fourteen Daily Audits Your Business Manager Should Make

1. From a control of income, the business manager (BM) reviews the daily receipt book that is prenumbered with carbon copy receipts.

2. He or she scrutinizes the checkbook to see that appropriate entries are made. These would include deposits, disbursements, adjustments such as bank charges, and other items. Overdrafting is avoided this way. A proper cash balance is maintained. However, only the doctor should sign checks to keep control of what the practice is buying.

3. The BM looks over the daybook and spot-checks for accurate postings from the daybook to account cards. Deposits from the daybook should be checked to see that full acknowledgments are made.

4. The BM sees that prenumbered charge slips are itemized for the service rendered and that they indicate the next appointment. (See Figure 1–1, a sample charge slip.)

5. He or she reviews color-coded medical records that have been removed from the active files. Your business manager may be able to avoid a potential problem by contacting the patient or learn of some error that has caused the patient not to return to your office. Anything unusual should be brought to your attention. Color coding is valuable in either numerical or alphabetical filing.

6. Monthly grouping files for paid bills let you or the BM look to the check register or the checkbook itself, for proof of when any particular bill was paid.

7. The BM brings you completed insurance forms. Always read insurance forms before you sign them. Don't let your insurance filing clerk hand-stamp them with your signature.

8. The BM keeps the six-day visual week-at-a-glance appointment book used in your office and observes how and for whom you are occupying your working time. He or she alerts you to expenditures of inequitable periods spent on less productive activities.

9. New patient information forms can be valuable sources of insight when the BM goes over them. After you have had a few contacts with patients, the BM's observations often will offer you insights into why certain individuals behave as they do.

10. The BM audits accounts receivable by reading the daily ledger maintained for each family instead of for single patients. The aging of delinquency is easier to see when you or the BM looks at a family's ledger. A clerical assistant has to determine which family member is to be credited with a payment if other than family account cards are maintained. Keep these ledger cards in a fireproof container.

11. The BM reviews billing and statements as they are being written.

FIGURE 1–1. CHARGE SLIP
In duplicate. One copy for patient.

No. 15885

YOUR NAME
ADDRESS
PHONE NUMBER

DATE ______

PATIENT'S NAME:
ADDRESS
CITY STATE ZIP

W: 1 2 3 4 5 6 7 8 9 10 11 12

O: ______ M: ______

YOUR NEXT APPOINTMENT IS:	AM
DATE TIME	PM

THIS MAY BE USED FOR
INSURANCE OR MEDICARE PURPOSES

DESCRIPTION	√	AMOUNT
COMPLETE HISTORY AND EXAM		
CONSULTATION		
ANNUAL PHYSICAL EXAM		
OFFICE VISIT		
OFFICE VISIT WITH INJECTIONS		
PHYSIOTHERAPY		
LAB ECG ☐ CBC ☐ UR ☐		
CHEM		
PAP ☐ RF ☐ FBS ☐		
BUN ☐ PBI ☐ TBI ☐		
URIC ☐ PT ☐ TC ☐		
CHOLEST ☐ BONE MARROW ☐		
OTHER:		
TOTAL CHARGE		
PREVIOUS BALANCE		
TOTAL AMOUNT DUE		
PRESENT PAYMENT		

PATIENT RECORD

AUDIT COPY

UARCO BUSINESS FORMS CHICAGO

E-Z-OUT®

12. The BM may occasionally listen in to telephone communications and to interoffice communications and report to you the ones of interest. He or she makes sure that buzzers and lights on phone instruments are in proper working order.

13. The BM makes monthly control audits of the dollar value of services rendered, the collection ratio, the office's collection ratio compared to other years, expenses incurred compared to previous years, the profit that results from expenses subtracted from income. Then your BM reports these statistics to you.

14. The BM evaluates collection procedures with delinquent accounts and decides if collection agency assistance is required.

HOW TO GET YOUR MONEY'S WORTH FROM A PRACTICE CONSULTANT

Your business manager may, as a result of various daily audits, bring news of a disturbing trend in your practice; perhaps growth has leveled off or even lost ground. An easy and established method of determining what is wrong with a practice that is not growing is to seek out competent assistance from the expanding specialty of medical management consulting. *Beware:* There is a limitation on how much advice or other help you can get from colleagues.

A management consultant may bring you expertise from observing a number of different medical practices in action. He or she can pass along dynamic advice that bridges the gap between the art of medical practice and the commerce of a smooth-running, thriving business. Management recommendations develop through specific application so that you can concentrate on medicine while your *business alter ego* works out the necessary but more mundane financial matters.

The medical management consultant will be both a specialist and a generalist. He becomes a specialist by limiting himself to your individual situation. At the same time he remains a generalist who applies his expertise to all the business needs of a medical practice. These will include your requirements as the buyer of insurance, the maker of investments, the payer of taxes, the user of supplies, the hirer of employees, the purveyor of services, the signer of contracts, the conductor of transactions, and the many other functions you have to perform in areas that take time and attention away from the practice of medicine.

In the past, hiring a professional management consultant was considered by some physicians as a kind of status symbol. Circumstances have changed that attitude today.

Because of the complex tax maze, corporate structures, rising operating costs and the third party involvement in medicine, you are forced to seek outside assistance. You must devote more attention to the business side of practice even as patients have increased their demands on the consumer side of medicine.

No physician can afford trial and error for solving practice management problems anymore. The professional practice consultant helps the modern physician make more vital business decisions with fewer errors.

Traditionally, management consultants have emphasized efficiency as an offset to rising costs coupled with tax preparation and tax planning expertise. Nowadays, his or her services have moved far beyond these narrow areas. The consultant does fee structure and expenditure evaluations, makes time and motion analyses of you and your personnel, and looks at every aspect in the delivery of medical care and the running of a practice as a business.

The best way to get your money's worth from a professional practice consultant is to have him initiate a total survey of what you are doing or are not doing every day, throughout your fiscal year. The consultant's services become most valuable when he does a complete medical practice management analysis of your office operation.

Responsibilities of the Professional Management Consultant

A professional management consultant comes to you with certain presumed duties and responsibilities. They fall into five generally defined categories:

A. Maximizing your earnings within the confines of your philosophy and the conditions under which you work.

B. Minimizing your concern with the business side of practice in order to allow optimum time for your attention to medicine.

C. Assisting with resource information for your entering into joint ventures, corporate structures, group practices, and other areas of business.

D. Working in liaison with other members of your business advisory team such as your attorney, insurance broker, investment counselor, accountant and others.

E. Generating a retention of your earnings for eventual retirement using such devices as tax shelters and various legal and strategic maneuvers.

The management consultant accepts these responsibilities in advance just as you accept in advance the obligation to keep your patient free of disease. The management consultant metaphorically is your coach while you are the quarterback who carries the financial football for a security touchdown.

Important: A consultant's job begins with your efficient bookkeeping system. If you don't have one already, this will be his first assignment.

Also, he assists in solving various problems that arise from buying and selling a practice or setting up a partnership or corporation. If you have a tax audit, he battles with the Internal Revenue Service. The consultant takes on the responsibility to keep income taxes current and to explain the tax consequences when you contemplate any business move.

Getting your money's worth from a practice consultant is accomplished in much the same way a patient would get his money's worth from you. The patient simply follows your advice. The management consultant generates advice from the strength and depth of dealing with similar problems under like circumstances faced by other doctors. You ply your profession, and the management consultant plies his. Both of you recognize that each has made an investment of time, money, and effort in getting the best training available. Just as your exposure to many patients has value for that single patient who wishes to get his money's worth from seeking your services, the consultant also acquires that same kind of exposure with many clients.

It is rare for any medical training to be accompanied by instruction in the art of practice management. You did not learn how to be a financial wizard or an office efficiency expert in the clinic or laboratory. You do need outside help for that kind of specialization just as you require outside medical consultants.

Is a professional practice management consultant expensive? Not in proportion to the amount of money you can save and earn from taking his advice. Besides, adjustments may be made.

> *Case in Point:* Fee adjustment took place between H. Peter Nennhaus, M.D. of Chicago and Charles H. Walsh.
>
> Dr. Nennhaus was attempting to establish his practice in cardiovascular surgery, one of the more difficult specialties to get off the ground financially. After seeing the numbers the doctor was generating from his practice, Walsh, the practice management consultant, voluntarily lowered his fee. The doctor accepted the adjustment with gratitude.
>
> As Dr. Nennhaus developed over the ensuing months and approached his gross annual goal, he became delighted with the way his practice moved upward. Without prompting, the cardiovascular surgeon came forward with the offer to return to the initial fee quoted by the consultant. It's a pleasurable circumstance not easily forgotten in one's professional life.

chapter two

Humanizing Patient Care Brings Big Dollar Earnings

You will discover that while the patient wants the best and most modern treatment available, he is also badly in need of the old-fashioned friend that a doctor has always personified and which you must continue to be. In his mind's eye, the patient sees you as in the old paintings or in his real memories—rumpled and kindly, roused from your bed at three in the morning to come to his home and pull him through a crisis. But . . . you will treat him in the clinic or the hospital whenever possible because the care you give is far better in those facilities. You will try to avoid night calls because you can diagnose better with your eyes open.

— Gunnar Gundersen, M.D., past president, AMA, Commencement address, Stritch School of Medicine, Loyola University, Chicago, June 7, 1962.

Patients are pressuring physicians for a return to the practice of humanizing medical care. More and more today, consumerist attitudes are having their effects on the relationship between doctor and patient. With the potential for national health insurance coming to fruition in this country, health care communication will have to get better. There must be some healing changes in the current delivery of medical service; otherwise, practice production will diminish and dollars will be lost for both patients and doctors. Holding onto much of your $250,000 gross income won't be a reality if you don't drift with the current of medical consumerism.

Case in Point: An internist in solo family practice in the heart of New York City, Marvin S. Belsky, M.D., encourages his patients to question his methods and motives at special "feedback" sessions for that purpose. The result is a welcome interchange between doctor and patient that inevitably leads to a deep, honest and direct relationship of genuine sharing and mutual participation.

Dr. Belsky calls his practice humanization technique the *Patient-Physician Feedback Group*. It is a biweekly routine part of his practice and not an experiment.

None of the meetings are gripe sessions or just accumulations of patients' complaints and condemnations. Rather they are attempts by people—the doctor and his patients—to find out how they may alter medical care from the treatment of diseases to the treatment of men and women—the "holistic" concept of health care.

Each feedback session differs. Belsky's technique increases his production and income by removing obstacles to strengthening the patient-doctor relationship. It gives patients a chance for input both collectively and individually. His method may be integrated into any practice or institution easily, because it transcends different cultural and psychological backgrounds.

"My approach aims at correcting defects in communication between a doctor and his patients," says Dr. Belsky. "That's necessary since a critical fault in the delivery of quality medical care comes from the gap in patient-physician communication."

The Belsky Technique Brings in $250,000 a Year

In an informal setting which disarms his patients' social conditioning, family conditioning, experiences with other physicians, and that certain ritual which they must go through during any doctor's office hours, Belsky conducts a group encounter session. Patients come by invitation prepared for a straight talk with their fellow patients and with their physician.

Belsky explained, "Twice a month, after the day's work is over, I sit in the reception room with my patients and we visit together. I am in shirt sleeves with tie loosened. We discuss our feelings—what they think of me as a person; our relationship; the office procedures; how to contact me in emergencies; my hospital affiliations; the nature of their health problems; education about medicine and its methods. They know in advance as part of my procedure that I meet with patients every other Thursday evening for a pleasant three hours.

"From each other we learn of our expectations and how they may be fulfilled," Belsky continued. "I inform them of patient roles and responsibilities and how to achieve them. In turn, I have received valuable critique and suggestions about my office setting, telephone appointments, office personnel, collection procedures, and general office policies. Also I learn about my patients' sources of health information, their fears relating to diagnostic examinations, tests and treatment and how their health habits have been influenced.

"I tell them about laboratory procedures, follow-up care such as prescriptions, diet, health habits, specialist referrals and hospital facilities and care. I tape record my feedback groups so I can listen later and analyze them for information," Belsky said.

One interchange during a Patient-Physician Feedback Group occurred when Belsky asked nine patients or family members gathered after his office hours: "What do you think makes a good patient?"

A young Spanish woman, answered, "A good patient is someone who obeys her doctor!" The others nodded their heads and offered supporting commentary.

Belsky followed that with, "Suppose your doctor gives you medicine that makes you dizzy? Would you continue to take that medicine?"

"Of course not," another patient said.

"But if you don't take the medicine, you're not obeying the doctor! Are you still a good patient?"

From this the patients learned that they have an obligation for mutual participation in health care delivery and that the patient must take care of his or her own health. He described the newer dimensions of patient care as opposed to the usual role of the active doctor and the passive, obedient patient.

Dr. Belsky has taken on the role of "country doctor" in the heart of midtown Manhattan in order to humanize his patient care and achieve a more productive practice. This creates happier patients and increased practice income. The internist raised his annual gross by 75 percent when word got around that he is a doctor who wants to hear about what patients are thinking. He now brings in big dollar earnings in the vicinity of a quarter million a year.

HOW TO OVERCOME IMPERCEPTION AND GET PATIENT FEEDBACK

Some physicians are quite perceptive about the feelings patients have. Others concern themselves only with their patients' physical conditions. Perhaps both types of patient needs, emotional and physical, are important to you and are perceived. But times are bound to arise when you and your patient do not seem to communicate effectively. Most often the problem will be one-sided—your patient thinks you know or understand or suspect more than you do and that you have some special knowledge to decode his feelings. At another time you may be less than the all-seeing being you are put on a pedestal to be—less than perceptive. A communication gap then will come between you.

The perception technique of "feedback," the kind that Dr. Belsky uses routinely, can prove most valuable to preserve the patient-doctor relationship. It is a technique we recommend you investigate to better humanize patient care in your practice.[1]

THIRTY BENEFITS FROM CONSTRUCTIVE PATIENT FEEDBACK

Constructive patient feedback will enhance your medical competence, because competence is intimately dependent upon communication and compassion. Where there is a lack of these two elements, competence has to be diluted, thwarted and aborted so that practice production inevitably suffers. Money is lost.

The many benefits of patient feedback build one upon another. Here is an integrated checklist that shows the benefits of feedback and how each builds on the one before.

Constructive patient feedback will:

1. Lower barriers to communication between the patient and you,
2. Lead to greater patient understanding of the medical world in which you work and what are your personal expectations in that world,
3. Contribute to increased patient cooperation,
4. Produce more patient satisfaction because your patient becomes aware of the procedures and processes you must utilize,
5. Cause less frustration for both you and the patient,
6. Save time for both of you,
7. Reduce patient turnover,
8. Let you know the patient's universe better,

9. Encourage your patient to express himself in a mood and setting that's friendly,
10. Provide certain information that lets you make practice management changes suggested by patients,
11. Make you aware of complaints and upsets before patient rancor sets in and a complete breakdown in relationship takes place,
12. Secure constructive criticism in an amiable atmosphere about consultants, office personnel, hospital personnel, collection methods, fee for services, and other mechanics of practice,
13. Allow for changes in consultant relations because of impingement upon patient acceptance and cooperation,
14. Have your patients learning from each other under your supervision,
15. Increase attention to a patient's therapeutic regimen,
16. Help to change poor health habits into better ones,
17. Promote social health goals and health maintenance on a personal basis,
18. Give patients the feeling that they are working with you in the health sector,
19. Make the patient understand that your practice problems are his problems too,
20. Give you a chance to know your own attitudes and feelings through the eyes of the recipients of your experience and training,
21. Tend to eliminate your being accountable to some bureaucrat who intrudes into medicine,
22. Enhance trust and confidence in you by your patient,
23. Attract more patients since you show such deep concern for them,
24. Meet the needs and demands of the American Hospital Association's "Patient's Bill of Rights,"
25. Fulfill society's mandate for the medical profession,
26. Adhere to the changing concept of medicine as being a team effort with the patient becoming integrated into the team,
27. Alleviate the pressure on patients to bring malpractice claims,
28. Offer more realistic expectations on the patient's part,
29. Act as a striking new modality for patient motivation,
30. Define in an experiential way a new role and a new responsibility for your patients.

We know that communication between you and your patients will provide an increasingly productive medical practice so that you can achieve a gross income of $250,000 annually. *This is absolutely realistic.*

By communication we mean the transmission of thoughts or notions from one of you to the other as well as from you to yourself. Self-communication, of course, takes place constantly when you think, emote, sense, evaluate and comprehend. Self-communication is basic to all communication with anyone, but it can be flawed at times.

Take for example the meaning of the term *pain*. From childhood memories of when a person was disciplined by parents that are carried into adulthood, to have "pain" may mean sharp smarting sensations and the components of fear, rejection, rebellion or resentment. The semantic understanding of pain sensations to you may be different than to your patient.

The same may be said of relationships. No environment, event, circumstance or object may be considered in isolation to either you or your patient. Everything is measured by conditions at the time. The occurrence of a person's pain and the amount of discomfort it gives will frequently vary with his personality pattern or his current environmental status. Relationships color semantic understanding.

> *Case in Point:* Voltaire, the great French author, philosopher, and apostle of free thought, met a downcast friend in an exceedingly dejected mood. The man announced that Voltaire should wish him a permanent farewell, for he was going to commit suicide that very afternoon. "Life no longer has any attraction for me," said his friend. "I am going to seek my fortune in the arms of the Gods. Goodbye, old friend." They shook hands.
>
> Voltaire was much shaken by this meeting. The following day, however, the two met again. This time Voltaire experienced a mixture of two emotions, anger at the false anxiety he was forced into feeling and relief at his friend's apparent continued good health. Voltaire questioned the fellow as to why he had not carried out his intention of the day before to commit suicide.
>
> His friend replied, "Since I spoke to you yesterday morning, I had a good bowel movement. Life is indeed wonderful today!"

As Voltaire, you, too, must be more careful not to project unconsciously your own referents and assume that your patient would use the same. Interpretations depend upon the individual's past experiences, past and present circumstances, drives and status at the moment.

Misunderstandings in your doctor-patient relationships can be avoided by making certain that your patient truly grasps, understands, and desirably responds to your projected words and thoughts. You have to almost step out of your skin so to speak in order to most humanize your patient care.

Someone has said, "Life is many things, it is food getting, shelter getting, hoping, arguing, aspiring, sorrowing; and in the center of it all, is the process of getting ourselves believed in and accepted."

To be a successful physician requires in turn the response, friendship, and confidence given by other human beings. When you provide fine medical service and combine with it frankness, kindness, and empathy you will be living up to the image the public has of a physician. It is the best use that you can make of your personality—the effect you have on other people.

SEVEN BASIC PERSONALITY TRAITS FOR A HUMANIZED PRACTICE

Seven basic personality traits influence your financial success in medical practice. Research has been carried out among postgraduate students in the health sciences by G. W. Crane[2] to select the doctor the students considered best of those they had visited during the course of their studies. The students were asked to write down the reasons for their choice. When results were tabulated the traits of humanization in medical practice through personality stood out every time.

Described in the order of importance listed, the seven traits of humanized practice were:

1. *Agreeableness.* "The doctor is cheerful, friendly and congenial." The attributes reflected by these personality traits are those you show through acts of courtesy, politeness and accommodation to your patients.

Important: One trick to enhance the agreeableness image is to keep a card file of personal information about each patient and his family so that you are conversant with affairs of interest to that individual. You can easily make him feel that he occupies a special position in your practice.

2. *Artistic Listening.* Without uttering a word, you can be more flattering to your patient, be he a day laborer or a financier, by facing the person, and listening attentively, and creatively. Listening is an art. It is an easy way to charm people and an almost certain method of creating a favorable impression.

Be Aware: Clay W. Hamlin, among the most successful insurance salesmen in history, once said, "About 90 percent of each of my interviews is devoted to listening. The quicker we give a man an opportunity to speak, the quicker we shall get the response we want. Let people talk; they really are thinking out loud."

3. *Persuasiveness.* The ability to convert a disagreeing patient to your way of thinking and to move him into a health program contrary to his conditioning is a major personality trait for practice success. Businessmen know that it is possible to win an argument and lose a sale—an ounce of suggestion is worth a ton of argument.

Crane says, "Guide me deftly to the decision you want me to make. Don't crowd, don't shove, just feed me ideas as fast as I can absorb them. If you can influence me to persuade myself, I'll sign."[3]

Therefore, avoid arguments and use your persuasive personality. Ask yourself this: "What do I really want from my patient? Do I want to win an argument and make an enemy, or do I wish to gain my point?"

4. *Compliments Must Accompany Any Criticism.* The tactful use of constructive criticism will get you more patient cooperation than will complaints and condemnations of actions. Negative criticism that aims a death blow at an individual's self-respect seldom works to your advantage. Instead, it places the other fellow on the defensive, makes him appear foolish in his own mind, and often accomplishes just the opposite of the desired effect.

Behaviorists have said that every course of action followed throughout life has been selected because it gives more pleasure than pain. Therefore, you must help your patient justify his actions before he carries them out. Let them give pleasure. That is where compliments come in. Use them first, before you offer criticism, no matter how valid it is.

5. *Mental Peace through Modesty.* Any of us will have little difficulty in thinking of acquaintances who have the fault of inflated egos and exaggerated opinions of themselves. Instead of letting others discover their underlying good qualities, they extol their own virtues at every opportunity. In so doing, these egotists arouse feelings of antagonism among most of those with whom they come in contact. Don't be one of those egotists.

To be one of the earners of a quarter of a million dollars in medical practice each year, present a front of mental peace and modesty. If you are content in your own mind, you will find it unnecessary to attract attention by exaggeration or egotistic statements.

6. *Associate Names with Remembered Faces.* One day, a young woman told her girl friend, "I don't think my gynecologist is really interested in me as a person. Even though he has taken care of me these last few years, he had to look at my chart to remember my name. Unfortunately for him, his assistant had slipped the wrong chart onto his clipboard, and he called me by the wrong name. Maybe I had better change doctors."

Vital: Your role as physician obligates you to give people nourishment for their self-esteem as well as for their physical health. Do this most effectively with warmth and interest by at least knowing your patients' names. No music is sweeter to a person than the sound of his own name.

7. *Find Traits to Admire in Others.* Sincerely and honestly tell of your appreciation for the many fine qualities that you find in other people. Be sensitive to patients, show concern and empathy, and use the spoken word to give a compliment.

The seven personality traits we have cited certainly are not new in their revelation. Often enough, however, even in their simplicity, they are overlooked. While what is needed comes naturally with social intercourse and social intelligence, sometimes a little more effort must be made in pushing yourself out of an introvertive bent.

Remember: You have to see the viewpoint of your patient.

Henry Ford said: "I am convinced by my own experience, and by that of others, that if there is one secret of success, it lies in the ability to get the other person's point of view and see things from his angle as well as your own."

THE TEN COMMANDMENTS OF HUMAN RELATIONS

The formula for making and keeping patients as friends might be considered a formula for human relationships in general. There are ten commandments:

1. *Speak to people.* A simple greeting lets the other individual know that you are not unfriendly and that you do, indeed, acknowledge his existence.

2. *Smile at people.* It takes seventy-two muscles to frown and only fourteen to smile. Take the easy way in this instance.

3. *Call people by name.* Anyone will be pleased and grateful to know that you consider his name important enough to remember and to use.

4. *Be friendly and helpful.* Remember what Emerson said: "The only way to have a friend is to be one."

5. *Be cordial and courteous.* Get into the habit of speaking and acting as though everything you do is a genuine pleasure. After a little practice it will be.

6. *Be truly interested in people.* Most individuals are deeper than the masks they wear and more interesting than you judge at first; just give yourself an opportunity to find out.

7. *Be generous with praise.* A pat on the back for something someone has done serves a double purpose. It makes that person feel good and it raises your own stature.

8. *Be considerate of others' feelings.* When you regard the consequences of your words or deeds the recipients will appreciate it and remember to someday return the favor.

9. *Be respectful of others' opinions.* Just as you prefer to have your say, let the other fellow express his views too. You don't have to agree with him, but on the other hand you might learn something valuable.

10. *Be alert to give service.* Be the first to offer help, to console and cheer. That is what true friendship for patients and other people really means.

Principles for Daily Practice

Translating the *ten commandments of human relations* into direct patient rapport is easily accomplished. Just guarantee that you adhere to the following principles:

- Set and keep appointments reasonably punctually.
- Maintain reasonable office hours.
- Explain all charges on statements.
- Explain medical problems of patients thoroughly.
- Periodically test and retrain aides to insure their top performance.
- Have adequate reception room space.
- Establish and use an appointment system.
- Provide adequate telephone answering service.
- Keep your fees fair.
- In a large group practice make sure that someone acts as the liaison between specialists.

PROVIDING PATIENTS WITH AN OFFICE POLICY

An office policy statement prepared for patients is just as vital as the one you prepare separately for office staff workers. A written office manual can be an extremely important document in the education of your patients. It will save your time by informing people in no uncertain terms just what are your practice rules and procedures.

Preparation of this information booklet can reduce 25 percent of patient telephone calls relating to questions about insurance, fees, emergencies, and a hundred other circumstances. Additionally, the office policy manual invariably improves patient public relations.

The American Medical Association has suggested what a printed office policy booklet could contain. Include this:

- Tell of the type of practice you run and what kind of medical coverage you offer.
- Tell about one physician covering for another in the case of absence for vacation, illness or medical meetings.
- Explain your policy regarding appointments and how far in advance the patient should call to make an appointment.
- Urge patients not to be tardy for scheduled appointments.
- Suggest how far in advance an appointment may be cancelled.
- Include office hours and days the office is closed.
- If house calls are made, say when.

By outlining your system of practice, you can avoid confusion and hard feelings among patients. For example:

- If you charge for telephone consultations tell how much.
- Do you notify the patient of his results from laboratory tests? Say so!
- Explain about your answering service and how messages routinely get through to you and that you reserve a special time for call backs.
- Give information connected with fees, billing and collections. By including a few words about fee schedules you can open the door to cooperative discussions, reduce the collection headache, and ease apprehensions mutually felt by the patient and you.

Include the AMA's booklet statement: "To all my patients: I invite you to discuss frankly any questions with me regarding my services or fees. The best medical service is based on a friendly understanding between doctor and patient."

Finally, include your office policy in regard to insurance and legal forms:

- List the fee for filling out forms, if you charge one.

- Point out that a cancelled check serves as a receipt for insurance and tax purposes.
- Assure your patients that no information will be released from your office to insurance companies or attorneys without the patient's written consent.

There is no particular format for writing patient information booklets of the office policy type. The AMA offers the following general format only:

(1) Use the "you" form of address in the copy instead of talking about "the patient."
(2) Write in a friendly and conversational tone and avoid the authoritarian approach even in those areas where you feel strongly.
(3) Explain your policies in terms of the patient's self-interest.
(4) Distribute the booklets only to established or known patients.
(5) Do not use the mass media to disseminate your policies.
(6) Work with a printer who will help you decide on booklet size, type style and method of reproduction.

Set the booklet in twelve-point size type and print it on durable stock paper. Perhaps you should translate your message into a foreign language if your practice includes a large number of foreign nationals. We suggest that you order only a six-month supply of booklets in the event you wish to make revisions to your patient office policy.

REFERENCES FOR CHAPTER TWO

1. Belsky, Marvin S., and Gross, Leonard. *How to Choose and Use Your Doctor*. New York: Arbor House, 1975.
2. Crane, G.W. *Psychology Applied*. Chicago: Northwestern University Press, 1937, p. 563.
3. Crane, Frank. "Ten commandments for salesmen." *American Magazine,* June, 1920, p. 152.

chapter three

Applying Secrets of Salesmanship Multiplies Patient Referrals

The Chinese laundry doesn't have to compete: it's competed against.

— C.M. Tan, *New York Herald Tribune*, Oct. 23, 1960.

A surgeon told a young intern, "I can teach you all you need to know in an hour to take out an appendix, but it will take five years of general surgery residency for you to learn what to do if something goes wrong."

The same thing is true in developing practice growth. New patient referrals come from recognition by professional peers and present patients who become convinced of your sincerity and skill as a doctor. Sincerity is the first requirement of selling and make no mistake; developing referrals is a study in salesmanship.

A good definition of salesmanship is that it is merely the act of converting people to your way of thinking. Perhaps the most important sale you can make is to sell *yourself* on the value of what you do. Then, what follows more easily is the selling of your services to others.

> *Case in Point:* Fletcher James Johnson, Jr., a cardiovascular surgeon in Nyack, New York, once was a bellhop at Kutsher's resort hotel in the Catskill mountains, a black basketball player from the ghetto carrying luggage. Today he is implanting pacemakers in some of the very same people he served as a bellhop. He alone can take all the credit, say "Look what I've done," and emphasize that he had to study in Italy and Switzerland to achieve his goal.
>
> Now he is making better than $250,000 a year, proof to himself that he sells services held in esteem by others. He admits to being "totally black." But the patients this heart surgeon attends to are looking for help. They are more interested in capability than in color. And his capability is paying off with Johnson's ownership of a beautiful home in the old Dutch hamlet of Blauvelt and a Lamborghini sports car whose production he supervised "in Italian, at the Factory," he says with a smile.

FRIENDLY COMPETITION IN MEDICAL PRACTICE

The basic drive for anyone in business—a physician is a businessperson like others who sell something—is to acquire a following as quickly as possible.

Friendly competition is the way this is done. A sizable practice that is large enough to provide the outlets for your energy and training will yield a sufficient financial return and give you personal satisfaction.

Friendly competition in medical practice stimulates enhancement of skills and growth of individuals among all doctors. Everyone benefits from intra-professional attempts at increasing practice activity. The dynamic impulse to grow is a common denominator among professional people. It will be a continuing concern for the major portion of your career, until such time as retirement persuades you to turn over the reins to the incoming generation.

While the development of your medical practice is initiated by your own determination and sense of competition, its rate of growth will be influenced by the degree of acceptance and endorsement of the community. The plaudits of your peers will provide one stimulus to growth. To a greater extent, however, you will have to rely on the willingness and loyalty of the patients who buy your services to refer other patients.

Important: If you are to gross an annual income of at least a quarter of a million dollars, you have to learn how to use ethical methods for more practice referrals.

TEN ETHICAL PRINCIPLES FOR MAKING MAJOR MONEY

Before we get into the specifics of how to develop more practice referrals, it is necessary to discuss principles intended to aid you in maintaining a high level of ethical conduct. Today, many professionals in the allied health sciences are advertising. Their standards are slightly different from the physician's, although M.D.s can legally advertise, as well. The propriety of conduct by which you govern your relationship with patients, with colleagues, with members of allied professions, and with the public is more stringent than others. Why? Because you have more power with people and should not abuse that power in any way.

There are ten principles of medical ethics, which were laid down by the American Medical Association before they scrapped them July 22, 1980, in favor of a simpler and looser code. Still, these ten principles do make acceptable guidelines for conducting yourself in an honorable way.

Here, in modified form, is an explanatory listing of those ethical principles.

1. Since the main objective of the medical profession is to render services to humanity with full respect for the dignity of man, you should keep the confidence of your patient, deliver a full measure of service, and apply yourself to his medical requirements.

2. Education is something that never ends for the physician. Consequently, you should try continually to improve on your knowledge and skill in order to benefit both patients and colleagues.

3. While it is mandatory to keep an open mind regarding new procedures and therapies, you should practice a method of healing founded on a scientific basis. Don't voluntarily associate professionally with anyone who violates scientific

principles but don't condemn out of hand something about which you have little knowledge or have merely heard rumors of negative results. When in doubt about a procedure, investigate it thoroughly.

4. The medical profession has imposed disciplines on itself to prevent illegal or unethical conduct of its professional members. Rules are set, laws laid down, and while they may be changed in accordance with the needs of the times, in general, these rules and laws should be followed. Sometimes, unfortunately, you have to expose a physician who is deficient in moral character or professional competence in order to safeguard the public.

5. While it is well established that a physician may choose whom he will serve, in an emergency you should render service to the best of your ability to anyone. Don't neglect any patient; give adequate notice of your withdrawal from giving care.

6. Avoid dispensing services under terms or conditions which tend to interfere with or impair your free and complete exercise of medical judgment and skill. Keep the quality of medical care at the highest level possible.

7. Don't sell anything except your own services. Limit your source of professional income to the sale of your knowledge and skill and keep your fees commensurate with two factors: the services you've rendered and the patient's ability to pay. Neither pay nor receive a commission for referral of patients. In an exception to what's been said, you can sell drugs, remedies or appliances only provided it is in the best interest of the patient and not for the sole purpose of making a profit.

8. You should seek medical consultation upon patient request; in doubtful or difficult cases; or whenever it appears that the quality of medical care you are giving may be enhanced.

9. Do not reveal the confidences entrusted to you in the course of medical attendance, or the deficiencies you may observe in the character of your patients. The exception is a ruling by law or because it becomes necessary in order to protect the welfare of the individual or of the community.

10. The honored ideals of the medical profession are your responsibility. They involve not only individual patients but also society as a whole. In short, whatever you do professionally and personally should be done for the improvement of the health and well-being of the individual and the community.

HOW TO GAIN ACCEPTANCE BY THE MEDICAL COMMUNITY

The principles of medical ethics for the physician are stringent, but in a kind of juggling act they can be reconciled with the principles of salesmanship. Combining the realism of salesmanship with the idealism of high morality will foster referrals that are the foundation of medical practice. A specialist who relies on referrals learns this early. Acceptance within the medical community is the first step.

This is important: Assimilation into your local medical community does not necessarily mean that you must lose your individuality. In particular, this assimilation will come about by your willingness to take on your share of the mutual burden. It entails fairly regular attendance at medical society meetings, a readiness to carry the load of committee work, and general compliance with the local situation.

Do this: We suggest that the new medical specialist should rub elbows with potential referring physicians whenever the opportunity affords itself. Don't be shy about contacting established doctors and giving as many details about your background and training as are called for. Don't overdo it, but lay out your skills at least once and in private with the doctor from whom you would like to receive referrals. Most physicians will react favorably to this approach, since they will likely remember the days when they had commenced practice and were hungry for patients.

Another million dollar action idea: Seek counsel from an older medical friend in the community. A well-established practitioner more often will enjoy talking about the program he followed in order to get established.

Follow up: Once a colleague becomes a referring physician you should log the referrals from that individual. This is the way to insure your constant review of the patients he has sent to avoid any breakdown or neglect of this source of business. All you must do is to keep a simple listing of the referral dates, patient names, and their conditions. Occasionally checking this list will remind you to discuss this patient's progress with the referring physician when you see him in the hospital halls. Such remembrance shows you really care.

One more thing: Not having the occasion to make an entry on the referral list of a particular physician means that it's time for your follow-up with another personal contact. Correct the cause of his inactivity in referring patients to you.

If you are a consultant: You should be involved constantly with sharpening your consulting skills. Be the perpetual student. Seek out and attend seminars relating to the specific area of your interest. Present programs whenever you can to alert potential referring physicians to your skills and knowledge. Regularly meet with other members of the profession to exchange problems and fresh ideas. Learn from the experience of others and offer them tips from your own experience.

Anyone who has had to build a fire in the fireplace knows the importance of bringing kindling to the flame. Your knowledge and skills are the kindling for flaming practice growth. Spread them around among your colleagues. It's the way to get patient referrals.

PATIENT REFERRALS FROM CERTAIN ACTIONS

Horace Cotton of Albemarle, North Carolina, an expert in medical practice management, identified percentages of things to do in order to gain acceptance by the medical community. Referrals come as a result of your taking the following actions:

Action to Take	Percentage of Response
Report back promptly regarding patients	33%
Be friendly with hospital colleagues	22%
Do your best to return referred patients	11%
All other areas of gaining acceptance	11%
Give scientific talks	7%
Offer the referrer an active role	5%
Teach in a hospital	4%
Teach in a medical school	3%
Make your availability known	2%
Publish scientific papers	1%
Entertain colleagues	1%
	100%

The Six Basic Ethical Ways of Getting Known

Each new contact is a potential source of patient referral, and there is no good reason why you should close any door which leads to more contacts with people. There are essentially six basic and ethical ways of getting known. They are:

1. Take an active role in local organized medical activity.
2. Participate enthusiastically in local civic work and service clubs.
3. Give speeches and write articles beamed at your own specialty.
4. Whenever you can, communicate with lay audiences in talks, articles, and books.
5. Attempt to get yourself a position in medical teaching.
6. Insert your listing where the public can find it when looking for a physician.

1. Running for office in the county and state medical societies will encourage referrals immediately. This is the height of taking an active role in organized medicine.

An encouragement of referrals also comes from your appearance on scientific programs and the writing of articles published in clinical journals that are related to your specialty. That way, you make yourself expert in the field by the fact that you must study more to give the talk or write the article, if for no other reason.

2. One Texas physician told us, "I've joined the Rotary Club in my town and not only made a lot of new friends but gained a flock of new patients. It seemed as if they were waiting for me. My specialty is urology, and the average age of my

fellow Rotary Club members was approximately fifty-three, a time when men begin to have urogenital difficulties."

We have to offer a precaution about getting involved in civic or service club work unless your motives are more than the desire to gather new patients. Club members will see through self-aggrandizement if your only purpose is to spread your name.

3. Articles you've written and had published in your specialty journal will draw attention from local physicians.

4. Lay audience appearances where you share your knowledge about aspects of your specialty serve two purposes. They build your ego to realize that you can communicate what you know, and they are bound to supply one or two patients out of each appearance.

Talks to lay groups are the means to reach the masses. It's good for them to get the information and good for you to spread the word that you know something. "I find that my office is always crowded after each such talk," said Alvin Carter, a Georgia family practice specialist. "I speak any chance I can to parent-teacher associations, unions, service clubs, women's clubs, and any similar groups. The listeners later call for appointments and not only do I get new patients from their hearing me but others who read about the talk in the local newspapers get the message too."

5. A fine ethical way to build a practice is from teaching in a medical school or hospital. When patients or potential patients find out about the teaching appointment, practice volume grows. They like to think that they are receiving attention from "the professor." It adds confidence to the people's confidence in your ability.

6. There is nothing wrong with advertising what you do provided that your ads are not offensive to colleagues. How can you know? Ask them! Times are changing and medical consumerism is making professional advertising in the media quite acceptable.

Case in Point: Before inserting a two-column, three-inch display advertisement in his local newspaper, Bartholomew Bruce Fang, medical director of the Alabama Eye Center, P.C. of Montgomery, visited the offices of several of his citywide colleagues. Fang was the only ophthalmologist who specialized in the Kelman Cataract Phaco-emulsification technique, and he wanted to inform the population. To avoid the danger of professional jealousy resulting in minor attacks on his happiness as a professional person, Fang told his fellow professionals exactly what the ad would say and actually solicited their agreement not to raise objections.

It was not Fang's intent to offend them by standing out from among his fellows and force them to question their own professional images in the eyes of the public. Otherwise, their response would not have been inward but outward against him. Subsequently, he got them to participate in the creation of the ad and got rid of the danger of peer group anger that could have had devastating consequences for him.

We don't recommend participation in community politics as a practice builder. Medicine and politics don't mix. While you may become known around town, it's probable that you'll lose more patients than you gain. Certainly, you should never take sides on public school issues.

Whatever you do in this public relations area, do it because you sincerely believe in the correctness of your action. Give something of yourself to the profession and the community as an aid to your fellow man. Benefits that you reap in return should be only incidental. They will come! Your attitude of sincerity will reflect itself in the eyes of those who see what you do, and it will be impressive.

THE EFFECT OF ATTITUDE ON PRACTICE GROWTH

Many patients look at their doctor as if he is a shining knight riding the white horse, or a pedestal-placed symbol of steadfastness. Although you may find balancing yourself on a pedestal an uncomfortable position to be in, some people do put you there. They expect you to be above such plebeian matters as asking for money. They anticipate your being stalwart in the town. Certainly they don't expect any businesslike attitude, but rather a friendly, open, interested one—in them.

The result is that a terrible disillusionment will set in for these pedestal-placing patients if you use too many business tactics in your various relationships. Pedestal pushers find this offensive, especially when it comes to your asking to be paid.

In our opinion, before you have your accounts receivable clerk dun for collection or turn an account over to a collection agency, it is incumbent on you personally to review the individual circumstances. Use common sense. Know with whom you are dealing and think about what the patient's reaction will be to your collection clerk's action.

We mention money and collections here because they reflect sharply on your image-building and practice growth. The one definite way you can ruin a reputation for competence and knowledge is to go after payment in a rough-and-tumble way.

On the other hand, the opposite attitude—pussy-footing—also plays havoc with expanding a medical practice. You can be too soft and easy. An attitude that says "I am a doctor and not a businessperson" may seem dignified, but it leads you down the road to wasted expenditure of energy for time and effort put in.

Another incorrect attitude is one that considers employees too expensive. Personnel costs are significant but the lack of assistants when they are needed, or the wrong person in the job, can hurt your image. A good employee draws referrals from patients, for she represents you to the world.

A so-called "ivory tower" attitude, one that implies "I am important," is dangerous to practice development. Often such an attitude does not consider the patient's feelings because arrogance is blinding the doctor.

Personal habits, for example, being a "swinger," have harmed many a physician. The playboy syndrome is unappreciated by people who are ill. We suggest that you have your cocktail when you get home and not in front of patients. Your moral reputation is exceedingly important to maintain. *Loose morals lose patients!*

A feeling of mature confidentiality should be the prevailing attitude in your office and outside of it. Prohibit yourself and your staff from discussing private matters about patients in any place other than within the confines of your facilities. Gossip is taboo under any circumstances.

An attitude of being a "goodtime Charlie" with frequent conventioneering or vacationing tends to move you farther away from practice life. Time away from the office or just not being available will cause people to stop and think before they seek an appointment. Your frequent unavailability to respond to their medical needs will lead some patients to say, "Oh, I can never reach that doctor; I'll have to find somebody else."

THIRTEEN QUESTIONS TO ASK ABOUT YOUR REFERRALS

To capture referrals you must review the humanizing aspects of dealing with people as was described in Chapter Two. In treating a patient, not only is the treatment the basic requirement, but you should go another step: listen with compassion to the individual's questions. Answer them clearly. Reflect an emotional involvement. Remember that you are dealing with the person's most important inventory—his health.

Therefore, we recommend that you ask yourself a baker's dozen of questions that can be instrumental in drawing new referrals from your patients.

Here are the thirteen questions to ponder upon:

1. Am I really worthy of the confidence implied in this referral?
2. Am I keeping up with my education as a physician?
3. How is my relationship with certain key patients, who are the referring people in my practice?
4. Do I adhere to the basic principles of medical ethics?
5. Do I humanize my care to the new patients referred?
6. Have I assumed a godlike image and do I demand that people accept my treatment advice as absolute?
7. Are my fees commensurate with others in my field?
8. How can I do a better job for my referral sources?
9. Do I have an enthusiastic attitude and an image to match?
10. Do I actively become involved in the interests of other people and thus broaden my horizon in general?
11. Do I convey a positive attitude?

12. Do I keep physically fit the way I advise my patients?
13. Do I stay healthy mentally and emotionally?

IS YOUR PRACTICE RUN LIKE A CHINESE LAUNDRY?

The practice of medicine offers people personal aid in the event of illness and health education as a means of preventing it. If the service offered a newly referred person is the same or less than he has gotten elsewhere or is higher priced, less efficient, and less personal, this new patient will feel little inclination to continue with you as his doctor. However, if, like the Chinese laundry, you offer a superior type of service or if the person imagines that he has had that experience, there is created the possibility of a great potential booster in that person.

Like the Chinese laundry, the successful doctor who gets many referrals from fellow physicians and his own patients will be giving good service at fair fees in an efficient manner. That is the fundamental way to develop more practice referrals.

There is no more potent advertising medium than the satisfied and enthusiastic patient who is a self-appointed press agent for you and who sets out to inform the community of your merits. In every practice there are these self-designated boosters who act as catalysts for the development and continued vigor of your practice. We have called these boosters "key" patients. They bring new people into contact with you. When you spot a key patient, cultivate him or her. It will be the best time investment you can make for referrals.

THE ABCs FOR STIMULATING MORE REFERRALS FROM KEY PATIENTS

A. Never lose sight of the importance of friendship. Provide empathy, warmth and cheer. One way is to remember a person's name and use it. The beautiful sound of his name makes an individual feel important and draws his attention. To accomplish this remembrance most easily, make a quick review of the medical record and the notes you've made on previous visits about the patient's personal interests.

B. Make some small talk for a minute or two to put the patient at ease. Use the information gleaned from a glance at his personal history. In other words, get friendly before you get down to business.

C. Devote all of your attention to the patient and don't let calls distract you from giving that full measure of time.

D. Appear to be relaxed and unhurried rather than very busy and preoccupied. It gives the patient a sense that he or she has received your undivided concentration.

E. If you really do have the time, escort the departing patient back to the reception room and bid a warm farewell. It will leave a lasting impression.

F. For anxious individuals who have some dangerous condition, give your home phone number to call in an emergency. People rarely abuse the privilege.

G. Whenever you can, offer a patient some little service or professional sample without extra charge. Especially make it a point to do this on the first visit.

H. Never refer to any of your assistants as "my girl." It detracts from her professional stature or yours and does nothing to instill confidence in the patient. Speak specifically about "Miss Jones" or refer to her by her occupation—the technician, the office manager, my administrative assistant, the nurse.

I. Make follow-up telephone calls about the patient's condition rather than waiting for the patient to call you.

J. Never correct any of your personnel in front of the patients.

K. Learn and use the principles of human relations we have suggested in Chapter Two.

chapter four

17 Ways to Shield Doctors From Devastating Malpractice Suits

> *One of the changes I would like to see made a part of every physician/client relationship is a contract, either a verbal or preferably an informal one-page written agreement wherein the physician acknowledges his secondary role and the client [patient] agrees that the major responsibility for his health rests with himself. This might shift the primary role in maintaining well-being on to the client [patient], where it belongs, and do a lot more than the PR campaigns and dangerous practices of defensive medicine to alleviate the malpractice insurance problem.*
>
> — Donald B. Ardell, *High Level Wellness*, 1977.

Are you a suit-prone physician or do you just deal with suit-prone patients? Medical malpractice claims across the country are growing; premiums for professional liability insurance are increasing; the ratio of physicians being sued is alarmingly disproportionate to the numbers in practice. In short, the medical profession is in a crisis situation requiring emergency attention. You may be the next victim of alleged malpractice—real or imagined in patients' minds—or feel its side effects.

ONE OF THE FIRST U.S. MEDICAL MALPRACTICE DECISIONS

The lanky Illinois lawyer picked up the leg bone of a chicken and held it aloft before the judge and jury. The bone had been broken, then knit together.

"The plaintiff says that his leg should have mended as perfectly as this chicken bone," said Abraham Lincoln. "But anyone can see that Mr. Fleming is no chicken. He's sixty years old."

The jury smiled appreciatively at the famed Lincoln wit. The plaintiff, Samuel Fleming, glowered in silence. He had broken a leg and it had not knit properly. Now he was suing two Bloomington, Illinois doctors for professional negligence and Lincoln was defending them.

"A lame leg is better than no leg at all," continued Lincoln, "and that's just what Mr. Fleming would have had if it weren't for the skill and loving care of his two doctors."

But despite his eloquence, Lincoln lost the case. Other local doctors testified in court that the splints had been applied incompetently. On the strength of that testimony, Mr. Fleming was awarded $700.

The case was the first medical malpractice decision ever rendered in the State of Illinois, one of the first in the entire country. Today, more than 130 years and two million malpractice cases later, the picture is quite different. If an identical case were to arise now, the plaintiff might not find it nearly as easy to get doctors willing to testify on his behalf and thus not receive a penny. But if he could get expert medical testimony and win his case, the award might well be 130 times as great as his counterpart received a century and a third earlier.

Those two factors—huge court awards for some claimants, nothing for many others—have combined to make medical malpractice suits the most emotionally charged area of law today. Almost nobody is satisfied with the way things stand. Nearly everyone is seeking clear, definitive information to clear up the malpractice mess.

HOW SPECIAL INTEREST GROUPS SEE IT

Each person looks at this terrible malpractice situation in a different way, depending on to which of the several special interest groups he belongs.

As the lawyers see it: Far too many malpractice victims go uncompensated, and the large awards being received by a few are just beginning to measure the economic and personal loss suffered by innocent victims of medical blundering.

As the insurance companies see it: A few avaricious lawyers are encouraging patients to sue at the drop of a scalpel and, by skilled theatrical tactics, are driving court awards up to impossible levels. The result? Professional liability insurance premiums are growing at a faster rate than any other medical practice expense. The average premium for a practice grossing $250,000 annually is more than $8,000. In fact, the malpractice insurance premium for a surgeon in California, where patients are often the quickest to sue, is phenomenal. It represents nearly 35 percent of the doctor's expenses.

As the doctors see it: The threat of malpractice litigation seems like a sword of Damocles hanging over our heads, by which one human error, one misstep—or one conniving, neurotic patient—can wipe out the earnings and reputation built up over a lifetime of devoted service.

As the patients who are disgruntled see it: Doctors are crooked incompetents who take the trust and confidence a patient starts with and exploits it. "Woe be the patient remaining unwary of his doctor's ministrations," they warn. This chapter will devote itself to confronting the malpractice warnings propagated by this type of disgruntled person and how you can avoid the situation's side effects.

EVERY FOURTH PHYSICIAN IS HIT BY MALPRACTICE CLAIMS

One thing all of the professional observers agree upon: The problem is getting bigger all the time. According to a study made by the American Medical Association (AMA), one out of every four physicians has been hit with a malpractice claim at some time during his professional career. "Professional liability claims are not limited to a small group of 'malpractice-prone' doctors," concludes the

AMA. "Our figures indicate that professional liability is the problem of the many, not the few."

Furthermore, it is not limited to only the 400,000 practicing physicians in the United States. The problem is worldwide. It is an interprofessional problem, too. A recent survey taken by the American Dental Association revealed that 10 percent of the 120,000 practicing dentists are sued each year. Proportionately, even more podiatrists are being sued than are M.D.s. An estimated 29,500 malpractice cases are now being brought to court every year, but the number of suits is no particular indication of how many malpractice claims are actually lodged. Thousands are settled out of court, and no one ever hears about them except the parties involved and the doctor's malpractice insurance company.

> *Case in Point:* Lawyers know that instead of concentrating on the question, "Was the defendant to blame as the cause of the patient's injury?" juries now ask themselves: "How much insurance is the doctor carrying?"
>
> Plaintiffs' attorneys usually ask themselves the same question. This was the case of Louis Amatono, a dermatologist in Provo, Utah. Suspecting malignancy, Amatono applied radiation therapy to a 74-year-old woman's mole. An infection developed, then a deep ulcerative condition exposing the bone. The patient required six months' hospitalization plus surgery and skin grafting by a plastic surgeon. When she had recovered, she sued the dermatologist for $1,500,000.
>
> What defense did the skin doctor have? Practically none. He claimed there was a confirming biopsy; the laboratory had no record of it. He claimed to have lost his own records on the case.
>
> Just when things looked blackest for him, the plaintiff's attorney discovered that the skin doctor carried only $50,000/$150,000 malpractice insurance. Though the plaintiff probably could have won the case in court, her attorney accepted a $100,000 settlement.

The word is out—when in doubt about a doctor, sue! Patients no longer sue as a last resort. They do it as a specific sign of their disgruntlement, and their lawyers take a "flyer" as a way to make some money with just a little paperwork and a few phone calls. Thousands of suits are started and then dropped for lack of proof. The practice of tort law is the fastest growing specialty in the legal profession. Some lawyers specialize in nothing else but the bringing of claims against doctors.

The question is which claims are justified. Doctors and lawyers are bitterly divided on this point. "In some localities, malpractice claims have become so frequent that any patient with a less than perfect end result is a potential malpractice claimant," said the late Louis J. Regan, one of the nation's leading medicolegal authorities. "If this alarming situation were evidence that the medical profession was becoming increasingly inefficient, then the solution would of course be obvious. But the blunt truth is that the majority of claims are without merit."

WHY PATIENTS SUE THEIR PHYSICIANS

We've said that patients sue their physicans because of their particular dissatisfaction with services. From our discussions with plaintiffs' attorneys, we have learned that patients think of suits as a kind of "green poultice" to salve their wounded egos, to settle grudges or avoid paying bills for professional services. Sometimes they do it to strike out against everyone because they are suffering pain and grief, of course, but that reason is the exception rather than the rule.

> *Case in Point:* In 1965, a convict sued the prison doctor who had examined him before the convict entered prison. The defendant had a lot of company because the prisoner sued everyone remotely connected with his imprisonment—about one thousand people.

> *Case in Point:* In the case of *Brawley v. Heymann* (191 SE 2d 366, NC 1972), Mr. Brawley, the patient, was having a biopsy taken of a lesion on his back by Dr. Heymann, a dermatologist. The patient fainted. The physician gave him a whiff of ammonia and Brawley said he felt better.
> Heymann turned away to put the ammonia back in the cabinet and Brawley rolled off the table and was injured.
> The patient sued. His allegation was of professional negligence, not a claim that the table was defective. The court held that the question of negligence should be submitted to the jury, which ruled in favor of the patient.

Another reason why patients sue their physicians is Americans' increasing awareness of how they can use the legal process to declare their rights as consumers.

We have warned that medical consumerism is on the rise. You would do well to understand better what the patient wants from you—and talk about it with him at the appropriate time.

ARE YOU A SUIT-PRONE DOCTOR?

A breakdown in communication between the physician and patient is a problem. Of 420 physicians who had been sued or threatened with a suit and were questioned by the HEW's Commission on Medical Malpractice in 1974, 37 percent named "poor communication between physician and patient" as the single most common cause of malpractice suits.

"The suit-prone physician," the commission said, "is one who cannot admit his own limitations. When he is confronted by a dissatisfied patient, he often neglects the patient by dismissing his or her complaint as trivial instead of making the patient feel less angry, afraid or depressed."

Research psychologist Richard H. Blum, in a study initiated by the California Medical Association to examine the causes of patient dissatisfaction and the prevention of malpractice suits, discovered that there are facets other than a strict injury-lawsuit relationship. One of them is the suit-prone doctor, who accounts for 25 percent of malpractice claims with unwavering regularity.

These suit-prone physicians are insecure with both patients and colleagues, and uncertain of themselves. Not only do they rely on the admiration of their patients but they also fear their anger. They are derogatory about patients as people and are bothered by their emotions, as well as their own.

In their medical work, suit-prone physicians are less likely to refer to consultants, usually keep poorer medical records, get along indifferently with colleagues, and probably make more actual medical errors. Some are sadistic, dishonest or psychotic.

CHARACTERISTICS OF THE SUIT–PRONE PATIENT

Loran F. Pilling, a psychiatrist with the Minneapolis Clinic of Psychiatry and Neurology, Minneapolis, Minnesota, provided an interesting insight into the particular kind of patient who provokes malpractice claims.

Pilling described the paranoid or suspicious patient who is fundamentally unable to trust anyone, especially somebody in an authoritarian role. The paranoid person remains aloof and distant. He or she may be the "shopper" who travels from doctor to doctor continually derogating the entire medical profession.

"These people are overly sensitive to any evidence of failure on the doctor's part," Pilling said. "The ability to trust, which is an essential feature of any social relationship, is not present. It is as if they must prove to themselves that the doctor is not trustworthy, and, in fact, intends to do them harm. By distorting reality, they are generally able to prove to themselves that they were right."

Pilling continued, "The proper management of these individuals is most important because everything done to them is interpreted as an attack on them. Although not generally dangerous, they often carry out litigation proceedings against their doctor that, although seldom successful, can cause a great deal of needless inconvenience. It is important in these cases to have objective evidence of organic pathology before physical treatment is instituted. Symptoms that mimic illness can be a result of the emotional problems these people are harboring."

The psychiatrist added that a somatic delusion as part of a paranoid illness may be bizarre.

Case in Point: A new patient who is quite paranoid has had life experiences leaving her convinced that people are not trustworthy. The woman's parents taught her that too—don't believe people—fend for yourself—always be on guard—take care! As a result, what you, as a doctor, plan to do and what she, as a paranoid, believes you intend to do are in contradiction.

As yet, you don't know that the patient is paranoid, and you believe that she has come to your office so that you can do *for* her. But what the woman feels is that you are there to do *to* her. Consequently, the two of you are not communicating, and you cannot recognize this because she is wearing a disguise over her paranoia. She has planted it in place quite firmly because if you get to know her, she is convinced, you will surely take advantage of her.

As a physician, you represent authority to the paranoid patient. Sitting before you, he or she feels placed in the most threatening of situations. The patient imagines that he is facing the lion in his den.

The paranoid attempts to disarm you with flattery: "Your receptionist was very polite. Your nurse seems efficient. Your office looks well furnished and pleasant. Your background music is soothing," says the paranoid. His or her implications are: "All these things mean you are a better physician than all the rest. That's something I think you want to hear, doctor, and I'm setting you up. I may sue you, so watch it!"

Pilling said that life for the paranoid person is a constant battle to protect himself against other people. An authoritarian figure is symbolic of them all. He can get back at everyone by damaging the symbol.

When the paranoid patient confronts a doctor who is new to him, he is compelled to get all circumstances going in his favor. It's his protection. Every self-preserving response he possesses will be brought into play.

The suit-prone patient thinks, "In my paranoic judgment, the best way to set you up, doctor, is to swell your head with praise. I'm good at setting people up. If your needs are strong enough, you will be vulnerable to me and I will have you as an authority I can manipulate."

Pilling warns, "If you fail to identify that paranoic person and go ahead and perform a potentially upsetting procedure on him, his unusually well-developed perception will recognize this. That's when he'll make his malpractice claim. His logic is: 'OK, you did to me; now I'm going to do to you.' It's the 'eye-for-an-eye' concept. You won't lose the court case, probably, but in my experience, every time you go to court it's a loss."

GUIDELINES FOR EVALUATION OF THE ANXIETY-RIDDEN PATIENT

Urologist Alvin Zolman of Atlanta applies a practical psychological control to prevent himself from ever getting into malpractice trouble. By using certain anti-anxiety guidelines, he approaches his new patient in just the right way and hasn't experienced a malpractice claim for the last twenty-two of his thirty years of practice.

The control involves taking a small amount of extra time to make patient personality judgments based on the Zolman guidelines that follow:

First, classify each new person who enters your practice. Write on a 4" × 6" card that you file in the patient's folder with your diagnostic and treatment notes. Attempt to classify the idiosyncracies of his or her character into categories such as the *introversion-extraversion-ambiversion* typology brought to prominence by Carl Jung.[1]

Record also the deeper psychological meanings and motivations which may underlie the new patient-physician relationship. You may change your personal judgments as your relationship progresses. If your judgment about the person does change, write a new index card.

Don't make these judgments lightly. Take time and extra effort. Run less; think more.

Here are the Zolman anti-anxiety guidelines:

Guideline One: The medical situation seems to provoke anxieties in people. This results in their irrational attitudes and sometimes bizarre reactions disproportionate to the reality of their necessary treatment. During medical care patients frequently are affected by a physiology of fear.

Guideline Two: An ill person's anxiety may be so severe as to compel him to take what appears to be a self-destructive attitude. For example, he may delay treatment until irreversible changes have taken place by the spread of disease either in the affected organ or in other parts of his body. In his discussion of anxiety, Freud emphasizes that it is essentially an affective reaction to danger.[2]

Guideline Three: Anxiety-preparedness in the face of any danger is a very adaptive reaction.[3] Thus, if a patient feels a sense of helplessness in the face of an inability to cope with it, he will find the situation traumatic. His anxiety emerges simply from ordinary medical treatment which has failed to produce improvement. The symptoms persist, as a result, and the sick person gets worse. His situation will now become serious. Prior to this, the illness may not even have been considered dangerous, but when the medicine currently in use does not work in an anxiety-ridden patient, the situation rapidly deteriorates.

At this point the patient's situation may personally affect the physician because the question of alleged medical malpractice is raised in the patient's mind. Either the sick person or his associates will suspect that the cause of his illness is being hidden by the physician, or they may suspect him of using inappropriate measures—out of incompetence or out of some kind of maliciousness.

Guideline Four: To ward off your own potential counterreaction to an anxiety-ridden patient's unnatural response to your therapeutic measures, you can institute a personal relations technique.

In some physicians, a personality maladjustment may cause them to undergo a reaction antagonistic to the real therapeutic requirements. One or the other may come over them like a wave: Either they feel that everything relating to this anxious patient is going wrong in some inexplicable fashion or, to the contrary, they find themselves becoming rigid and acting ridiculously calm toward him. The personal relations technique we will suggest can have you take stock of what your own reaction is.

The Personal Relations Technique

In daily practice at the day's end, we suggest that you evaluate your response to each patient's relationship with you. We call this technique the *evening evaluation*. It requires that you go down the list of people you've attended that day and check for some irregular behavior on your part toward a person. As you think back through the day, flag his personality card with a red, metal "fire signal," such as the Crimpgraf® plastic inserts.

When you see this fire signal during the patient's next visit, read his personality card again and put into practice the ten-point checklist that we will describe in a later section in this chapter.

The notations you made on the patient's personality card will help you to act in a more sensitive, less offensive and more accepting manner toward his particular characteristics. Make a studied effort to comfort rather than to upset the patient. Calm his anxiety.

We believe that the physician who is mature and capable of healthy social adjustments will have no trouble in making a sensible evening appraisal of his relationship with patients and taking necessary practice management steps. It will eliminate your getting sued out of anxiety felt by a patient or his family. For whatever reason some patient gets peeved, it won't be from suffering an anxiety reaction that produces traumatic neurosis.

Case in Point: Using these Zolman guidelines, Everett Jackson, another urologist in Washington, D.C., was able to make drastic cuts in the cost of his clinic's malpractice insurance payouts. With six physicians following the guidelines, there has been only one claim among them in eleven years in the Jackson Clinic.

THE REAL REASON PATIENTS SUE DOCTORS

While we have described the paranoic patient as possibly the most common suit-prone patient, the second most frequent source of malpractice claims comes from the anxiety-neurotic.

Anxiety reactions that produce traumatic neurosis cause this suit-prone person inordinate misery with fright, apprehension, and an enveloping sense of catastrophe.

Case in Point: One patient, a college girl who eventually brought suit, reflected acute anxiety in frequent physiological reactions: Her heart pounded; her breathing became irregular; she perspired excessively; her limbs trembled. The physician had to administer a drug for rapid sedation as the only means for the girl to escape from panic. This kind of patient is the constant victim of gnawing anxiety and tension and the potential plaintiff in a malpractice action against her doctor.

Why? We have previously mentioned that the offended patient's secret relief valve for the internal pressure of anxiety neurosis is to punish the doctor. You, the physician, after all, are the personal representative of an offensive health care delivery system. It is a system that creates resentful patients forced to undergo a thousand humiliating tortures and masterful insults. "Go into that room and take off your clothes," says your receptionist or nurse. Important people become unimportant patients. They lose cherished identities and become nothing more than so many bodies to be prodded and probed, stuck and catheterized. Our culture forces sick people into social inferiority—cases to be studied by the "superior" physician-scholar.

No wonder the anxiety-ridden patient becomes besieged by traumatic neurosis. He or she lets fantasies run free as frames in a movie film. The patient acts the role of long-suffering protagonist. And who is to play the antagonist?— "Black Bart, M.D."

Should some kind of health care accident or problem with the treatment occur, the frustrated, anxious and neurotic patient easily interprets this as a sign of the doctor's lack of personal interest or lack of professional competence. A medical malpractice suit will be the invariable result.

THE TEN-POINT PATIENT CHECKLIST TO PREVENT MALPRACTICE CLAIMS

You can shape your personality to match the patient's in the same way that you would develop a flabby muscle. Exercise it.

We recommend your use of a ten-point checklist to stop yourself abruptly and make you think. See if you discover any "no" answers to the following questions as you are examining or treating your patient:

1. Am I listening to the patient and not merely remaining silent while he is speaking? Am I giving him my undivided attention?
2. Am I avoiding abrasiveness as I respond to questions or give advice? Am I using gentle persuasion instead of argument?
3. Am I complimenting the patient first before I tactfully offer constructive criticism?
4. Am I freely giving the patient credit for following directions correctly and making my job easier?
5. Am I showing him respect as a person by being interested in him personally rather than in his condition?
6. Am I making an honest effort mentally to exchange places with the patient so as to understand his anxiety?
7. Am I nourishing his self-esteem by calling him by name?
8. Am I speaking in terms he can easily understand but which are not beneath his level of education?
9. Am I offering a constructive therapeutic plan that will likely restore him to health?
10. Am I giving the patient a choice?

THE MENACE OF PRACTICING DEFENSIVE MEDICINE

Supreme Court Justice Taft said, "A physician is not a warrantor of cures. If a failure to cure were held to be evidence, however slight, of negligence on the part of the physician or surgeon causing the bad result, few would be courageous enough to practice the healing art, for they would have to assume financial liability for nearly all the ills that flesh is heir to."

Of course, if the patient wakes up in a hospital bed the morning after an operation and hears a watch ticking where his gallstones used to be, he'll have good reason to suspect that some butterfingers was hovering over the operating table.

Counselor Melvin M. Belli, the patron saint of malpractice plaintiffs and the devil incarnate for the doctor defendant, said, "The malpractice situation has become so bad—especially in my home state of California—that something should be done about it. The courts actually are breaking down where malpractice law is concerned. Many jurors just won't sit on a malpractice case; many who do sit carry deep prejudices against dentists and physicians."

Belli points out that many jurors feel: "All doctors are no damned good; all doctors protect one another; medical fees are so outrageous that doctors should pay through the nose for their mistakes." Physicians know of this attitude, and the result is that they are practicing defensive medicine. This was proven by the New York State Senate public hearings in 1970 which elicited testimony showing a mercurial rise in malpractice suits. Potentially hazardous modes of treatment, though sometimes appropriate and life-saving, were bypassed by suit-shy health professionals who feared the legal consequences.

Attorney Belli's conviction and the findings of New York State are in contrast. The legal system is working not only against physicians but also against the public interest. Patients are getting less than perfect medical service because of the harassment of physicians. Defensive medicine has permeated American medical practice.

Leroy Lavine, M.D., attending physician in charge of orthopedic surgery at Long Island Jewish-Hillside Medical Center, New Hyde Park, New York, believes that defensive medicine is being practiced broadly. He said, "My impression is that there are many more consultations, X-rays and tests. I think defensive medicine is not limited to those who are sued most often. The medical men are doing it more and more, as are pediatricians. It may have started with the specialists who were sued the most, but everyone is aware of what's going on and everyone is thinking in those terms.[4]

Most physicians acknowledge that defensive medicine is a complicated problem, without easy solutions. One solution might be the elimination of the attorney's contingency fee. Other solutions could be "no fault" insurance funds, similar to present automobile insurance, or closer monitoring of less competent practitioners. The best solution, however, may be compulsory arbitration between the disgruntled patient and the defendant physician.

Should We Arbitrate Malpractice Cases?

The arbitration of complaints by patients of alleged malpractice by their physicians is an idea whose time has come. There are city- or county-wide arbitration programs in about thirty states. The American Arbitration Association (AAA) says that medical societies in a dozen states are now inquiring about statewide programs. "There's no question that interest is at an all-time high," says lawyer Irving Ladimer, special counsel for AAA health programs.

There is much to commend this approach to limiting the malpractice suit problem. For one thing, it is swift; settlement by arbitration may take an hour or a day, whereas a court case can drag on for weeks. Arbiters can hear the case rather promptly, while many malpractice suits may languish on court dockets for four or more years.

The arbitrators, who usually include physicians and trial lawyers, generally know a good deal about medicine. Their decisions, therefore, are less likely to be quirky than those of a jury; certainly the arbitration panels are less vulnerable than juries to the emotional appeal of silver-tongued lawyers.

For you, binding arbitration should be especially attractive because it leaves little room for appeal. Then, too, there is no intimidating publicity that might force you into a settlement you really don't believe is worthy.

The lawyer representing the plaintiff will find arbitration advantageous as well. He will have less expense out of his pocket, and less work. For the plaintiff, there is the opportunity to push a pint-sized claim. Nowadays, says attorney David M. Harney of Los Angeles, it costs $12,000 or so to press a malpractice suit, so suing for less than that is a losing proposition.

The insurance companies should like arbitration, since there is the chance of smaller, more reasonable awards. Arbitrators are not in the habit of handing out money for a patient's "pain and suffering."

Your attorney can tell you how to go about using the arbitration setup to settle patient grievances. In our opinion, this is absolutely the most effective way out of the malpractice mess in which doctors now find themselves. We suggest that you have your patient sign a contract to arbitrate any disputes at the time you get his informed consent to undergo any procedure. This is not an unprecedented action. A medical group in California consisting of 160 physicians and 400 other personnel, known as the Ross-Loos Group, which furnishes prepaid health care to more than 90,000 subscribers, has since 1930 required subscribers to accept binding arbitration as part of their contract.[5]

Case in Point: In one case that involved the Ross-Loos Group, *Doyle* v. *Giuliucci* (401 P 2d 1, Cal 1965), the contract to arbitrate was held to be binding. A child who had allegedly been injured by negligence of one of the doctors in the group was represented by her father. First he submitted the claim to arbitration, but changed his mind and prior to the arbitrator's decision he filed a suit. The child claimed that since she had not been a party signatory to it, she could not be bound by the agreement to arbitrate. The trial court held that the child was bound by the contract and the California Supreme Court held that the father did have the authority as her natural guardian to enter into a contract for the child's medical care. This bound her to arbitration. The court further held that the provision for arbitration was not an unreasonable restriction on the minor's right.

PREVENTING EXCESSIVE COURT AWARDS WITH THE MEDICAL MALPRACTICE ACCIDENT FUND

Fifty years ago an employee had to prove that his accident was caused by the employer's negligence, and that he did not contribute toward the mishap in any way. Justice was slow, erratic and uncertain at that time. Then, one by one, the states began enacting workmen's compensation laws, scrapping the whole theory of negligence and guilt as a basis for awards. "No-fault" automobile insurance has followed this pattern, as well. We recommend that the malpractice laws follow these same guidelines.

The laws recognize that industrial accidents are inevitable and should be compensated for, no matter who is technically responsible. The laws set up standards as to how much the injured employee should receive for lost wages, how much as recompense for the injury and disability, with a definite dollar amount for the loss of each phalanx of each finger. Deciding the amount of an employee's award is primarily a fact-finding job performed by impartial workmen's compensation examiners, without any stigma of blame, shame or guilt falling upon either of the parties involved.

How the Medical Malpractice Accident Fund Works

The same sort of approach can be taken with medical malpractice claims. The program we envision could work something like this:

Case in Point: In place of your malpractice insurance premiums, you might contribute to a medical accident fund. Patients also contribute a few cents to the fund for every dollar in doctor bills that they pay. It would be an addition to the bill and plainly marked as such. The collected money would be turned over to the Medical Malpractice Accident Fund by the physician exactly as he pays Workmen's Compensation premiums now.

Anyone who suffers an untoward medical result, whether or not caused by a physician's negligence, might make a claim against the accident fund. An expert panel of doctors and lawyers would decide whether the claim is justified and, if so, what should be the award.

The differences between the plan we propose and the present system are substantial.

Now, an aggrieved patient lodges a legal action. With our system, he would be filing an insurance claim.

Now, the amount of his benefits are decided by the skill of his lawyer and the emotions of a jury. By our fund system, the basis of his compensation would be from fixed standards.

Doctors have little reluctance to give medical evidence in workmen's compensation cases now, and they should have no more reluctance with our system for determining medical malpractice, later. They won't be branding a colleague a fraud or an incompetent or taking sides. Rather, and most important, our plan would recognize that a doctor can make a mistake without being careless. He can err in judgment without being incompetent. He is able to use new and daring therapy to save a life or limb without being labelled a "quack." Our plan frees him to do that.

Certainly our proposed Medical Malpractice Accident Fund is better than the present system wherein only some of the medical cases caused by accidents, and not necessarily the most deserving, are ever given compensation.

We believe it is better not to pit one doctor against another in court and ask a jury of six or eight or twelve people, good and true but medically ignorant, to decide which doctor is right and by how much. A fund set aside for medical accident compensation would take the emotionalism out of malpractice and clean up the present mess.

REFERENCES FOR CHAPTER FOUR

1. Jung, C.G. *Psychological Types*. New York: Harcourt, Brace & World, Inc., 1923.
2. Freud, S. *The Problem of Anxiety*. New York: H. A. Bunker, 1936.
3. Mowrer, O.H. "A stimulus-response analysis of anxiety and its role as a reinforcing agent." *Psychological Review* 46:554, 1939.
4. Gordon, Alex. "Practicing defensive medicine." *Physician's World* 2: 35–37, March 1974.
5. Rubsamen, David. "The Experience of Binding Arbitration in the Ross-Loos Medical Group," Appendix, pages 424–449.

chapter five

Picking the Medical Practice Formation That Reaps A Quarter-Million-a-Year

There is always serendipity. Remember the Three princes of Serendip who went looking for treasure? They didn't find what they were looking for, but they kept finding things just as valuable. That's serendipity, and our business is full of it.

— George Merck, pharmaceutical manufacturer, November 3, 1952.

Various benefits evolve from the different structural forms for medical practice. Some bring an easy quarter million annual income; others provide more free time. Don't choose yours by serendipity.

The decision as to what financial form of practice to choose is much too important to let things fall where they may. The circumstances of practice life are going to affect your happiness and health for a long time. Therefore, make a comparison and lay out the advantages and disadvantages of the four forms of practice structure.

Case in Point: In July 1976, Richard White, M.D. of Davis, California, took down the shingle from his office door. He was leaving the private practice of medicine. Medical practice serendipity had taken its toll of one more victim.

At age forty-eight, Dr. White finally concluded that any fun and interest for him in patient care had been removed by the high costs of malpractice insurance, the third party insurance intervention, and the singleness of service delivery expected. The undercurrent of medical consumerism had finally gotten to him.

The group in which this physician participated was abandoning many of the aspects of medical care that he enjoyed the most—surgery, obstetrics, and the handling of complicated therapeutic problems which required some concentrated and collective thinking. Now he had become a way station between his patient and the specialist—a kind of diagnostic traffic cop—and Dr. White did not want to send patients elsewhere anymore.

"I'd go to work, but I'd live for the weekends," White recalled. "It got boring. I had become just a talking and listening doctor." Serendipity or his own calculated planning and discovery led the physician to leave medical practice and to seek a position in industry.

Today Richard White is assistant medical development director for E. R. Squibb & Sons, the Princeton, New Jersey pharmaceutical manufacturer. He has become a member of an elite group—6,000 full-time corporate M.D.s in the United States. They include 1,500 physicians who work in the pharmaceutical field and about 1,000 who are insurance company medical underwriters and claim consultants. The rest are "occupational medicine physicians" whose job is to check out everything pertaining to employee health, industrial safety and product safety. Another 11,000 physicians serve part-time in similar roles.

MOTIVATORS FOR JOINING CORPORATE MEDICINE

The full-time occupational physicians usually drift into corporate medicine from military medicine, public health service, the ranks of the part-timers or from those private practitioners like Dr. White who become disillusioned with unpleasant conditions growing more prevalent in the rendering of patient care. White's prescription for curing his ailments of unhappiness with certain aspects of medicine was a change from one structure of medical practice to another. Might that be a prescription for you too?

Two motivators tend to make the corporate structure more attractive:

1. The money is steady and respectable with hours that are reasonable. The average annual income is $80,000 a year with no practice expenses. It's all yours to share with the Internal Revenue Service.

2. In industry there are often opportunities to practice preventive medicine with no limit to what can be done for patients simply because they don't have to pay for the care.

Overshadowing these motivators is the desire of particular physicians to get away from the various hassles of direct one-on-one patient care.

Many doctors are fed up with or confused by the serendipity of medical practice structure. Leon J. Warshaw, chief medical director for the Equitable Life Assurance Society of the United States, said, "I get calls every week from doctors who are interested in a change. They want to get out of the rat race of private practice."[1]

MIGHT YOU BE A SOLO COUNTRY DOCTOR?

Is the sophistication of industrial medicine for you? Maybe not! With so many rural communities looking for doctors these days you might be keen to bring the blessings of modern medicine to the fine, hard-working folk of a farm community. You could select a small town with no physician for miles and perhaps set up a little office in your home. Does that sound appealing?

It is likely that the townfolk will welcome you, even set you up, and after a while expect you to spend all your energies taking care of them. Of course, they may frown on any extracurricular activity for you except the practice of medicine. That's what you went to school to do, right?

Some communities feel they own their doctor and that he ought to be available constantly. Rural physicians affirm that many doctors either die young or are driven away or heroically get used to being roused from slumber at any hour of the night.

Case in Point: One country doctor, Austin P. Marmaduke of Swayback, Missouri, described his experiences as a solo practitioner. Marmaduke lives in an old house with many outside doors, one to the office and the others to his family's living quarters. No matter how late it is, patients beat on the doors as if they are drums—on whichever door they chance upon.

The entire household, his wife and four children, not uncommonly are awakened at 3:00 A.M. by a patient's banging, whistling, and shouting. Typically, Marmaduke hears calls such as "Doc! Hey Doc—wake up and git dressed! Elsie's havin' her baby any minute and you gotta git there!" Sometimes it is a job for the doctor just to locate which door is being pounded. He says he loves his patients though.

These same doors are occasionally entries for uninvited dinner guests. The doors are never locked during the day. The friendly country folk will come into the house unexpectedly and unannounced at any time. They arrive even when Marmaduke's family is eating. Patients are not shy about sitting down for a bite to eat without waiting for an invitation and proceeding to describe their physical complaints. The doctor doesn't mind because his patients are like members of the family.

Once Marmaduke was home alone, taking a shower, and a country stranger strolled into the front room downstairs looking for medical attention. He called, "Doc—hey doc, where are yuh?" The physician called back that the man should take a seat and he would see him as soon as possible. The next moment the new patient walked into the bathroom and at once began to shout his long list of symptoms over the sounds of splashing water. This was very amusing to the physician.

Bill Collections Are Difficult in the Country

Country folk consider the doctor a part of their family, as we mentioned. Consequently, it seldom enters their heads to pay him. Monthly statements for services rendered may be looked at as so many greeting cards. "How nice to hear from Doc again this month," they say. If he should attempt to collect payment, it is likely to be an action that antagonizes some people.

Solo practice in the country or in a medium-sized city or elsewhere has its rewards and disappointments. Just what they are will be determined in part by a basic lingering drive to attain what is important to you in life.

To some physicians, this may be having many patients as friends, and friends as patients; to other M.D.s it may be having a lot of money without patients necessarily being friends. In any practice structure you could find that economic security and personal life style will sometimes be in conflict. You may have to choose between making $250,000 a year or having 250,000 friends in a country region. More often you'll make $60,000 of gross income to go along with all those friends.

The Benefits of Solo Practice

Independence of thought and action are the most important advantages of solo practice.

• A single practitioner does not need to deal with someone else's decisions about the manner of his practice and the expenditure of practice time and money.

• The solo physician will experience less harassment by the Internal Revenue Service—there are no partners to involve him or her in a joint audit.

• Solo practice gives you the chance to be more humane. You can be a friend and advisor to patients without worrying about whether you are keeping up with your end of production in a partnership group or professional service corporation.

Certainly, money is important, but maybe the quarter million annually that we talk about as a goal does not turn you on so much. Having patients as friends may be far more important. You can carefully discuss the diagnosis and prognosis of problems with them using lay terminology. You can answer all their questions. Many people today feel dissatisfied with their medical care because they get too little information from some doctors.

Every patient has five basic questions he wants answered:

1. What is wrong?
2. What caused it?
3. What should be done about it?
4. How long will it take to fix?
5. What will it cost?

Being in practice by yourself affords you the opportunity to take time and substantially answer these questions. You can mold patients—create satisfaction. Businessmen long ago realized the importance of winning the good will of their customers and their communities.

The largeness of some medical structures has not allowed physicians to retain the respect and affection of their patients and the public. The doctor in solo practice, on the other hand, has a golden opportunity. He can adopt and make use of a public relations philosophy through building human relationships as we discussed in Chapter Two.

The Disadvantages of Solo Practice

• The main disadvantage of solo practice is that there is no sharing of responsibilities with somebody else.

• You are required to secure outside coverage while away from the office for a length of time.

- There are no death, disability, or retirement benefits as with working in a group.
- If there is no work from you, the practice income stops.
- The highest cost of working solo is probably the burden on your health. If you are incautious enough to overreach in patient care and take on more of a load than you can handle—being constantly on call at night and on weekends—your survival will be in question.
- Family life encroachments will occur too, and you'll have less time to live a normal home life.

Case in Point: Family practitioner Walter Glumby of Port Arthur, Texas was truly in love with the practice of medicine, but he had total loyalty to his family, as well. He was of a frame of mind, like Marcus Welby, M.D., not to cheat his patients on time and attention. At age forty-seven Glumby had forgotten how important it is to go out and play tennis or golf and to charm his wife, although he loved his family and life itself. Still, he was denying himself the beauty of marriage, seeing his children grow up, and the camaraderie of family fellowship. He was in conflict between two loyalties.

This family doctor was burning himself out, working eighty hours a week, being absolutely committed to his patients. He said to his wife and children, "I love you very much, but these people need me. They rely on me, and I feel I must serve humanity with my whole being." Glumby died of a heart attack soon after making that statement.

Advice for Surviving Solo Practice

So, there are pros and cons to solo practice even as the numbers of single doctors are diminishing. Yes, rugged individualists are fading away like many old soldiers. However, Robert D. Gillette, M.D., a general practitioner from Huron, Ohio, suggests that there are ways to make solo practice work more effectively and without burdens or encroachments. Dr. Gillette says, "Solo practice need not be a man-killer. Let me pass on some of the things I've learned about how to survive."

The following is what Dr. Gillette suggests:

Roll with the punches. Every phase of human endeavor has its frustrating moments, and the practice of medicine is no exception. If your life as a doctor is to remain pleasant, you need certain escape valves.

1. Accept people for what they are. There's a little stupidity in all of us, and it does us good to acknowledge our human imperfection.
2. Laugh a little. Most doctors take themselves too seriously.
3. Find ways to let off steam. This is an individual matter, and each of us must find his own solution. It could be golf, poker, gardening, or perhaps a rousing game of cribbage.

Don't let patients run your practice. With experience, a doctor learns to tell the difference between a manipulative patient and one with legitimate problems. The mother who calls you about a child with a 105-degree fever has a legitimate claim to your attention, but the one who phones during off-hours requesting a refill of her old tranquilizer prescription might be trying to manipulate you. Don't let her get away with it. You don't have to be nasty; just tell her you can't give her a refill without reviewing her chart, and ask her to call the office for an appointment. Patients can learn more mature ways of relating to their doctor if he will politely indicate what he expects of them.

Cut out the frills. There's no general agreement among medical men as to what parts of practice are superfluous. You'll be a better doctor and find your practice less of a drag if you concentrate on the things you consider important. For example, if you're successful in treating obesity, then stick with it, but if you find this an unrewarding area of practice, don't waste time on it.

Unload a few patients. There are occasions when a patient and a physician just don't get along. In most cases, the patient finds another doctor. Occasionally, you may wish to nudge things along by suggesting that the patient either do things your way or go elsewhere. Where? Many communities have a few doctors who aren't busy. Find out who these people are in your community, and send them your excess patients.

Why Solo Practice Will Endure

More than 50 percent of medicine is practiced in partnerships and groups. Professional group associates fulfill the common goals of enjoying more free time, increased earnings, greater efficiency of operation, use of better facilities, retirement benefits, buildup of definite estate values, upgraded practice skills, and built-in reliable consultants. How can anyone beat those benefits by practicing alone? It is true that you cannot surpass those advantages by much except that group practice physicians may forget one thing about the art of rendering medical care: Practice involves the patient and not just sophisticated machines of science.

Solo medical practice will endure, as we have said, because it gives you the opportunity to be humane—to listen and advise.

> *Case in Point:* A family physician in Weirton, West Virginia, Ray S. Greco, says: "Medicine is beset from within the profession and without by charges of inadequate attention to patients' needs. From all sides we hear demands for a return to the physician-patient relationship idealized by our grandparents, in which doctors not only attended to broken bones and infections but also did what they could to patch shattered egos and bolster confidence."
>
> Dr. Greco practiced as a family physician for a few years and then entered a psychiatric program for primary physicians given by the Staunton Clinic in Pittsburgh; he then returned to general practice.
>
> In contrast to Richard White, who left private practice because he had become "just a talking and listening doctor," Dr. Greco says that his psychiatric training reduced "my fear of listening, which permitted me to enjoy listening. I now use time more effectively, making quicker and more precise diagnoses.

This enables me to make more specific treatment plans and to have more confidence in what I am doing than I had before."

JOINT VENTURES IN MEDICAL PRACTICE

A joint venture with other doctors in a professional partnership or medical corporation provides a big benefit in that each doctor can be delegated separate responsibilities. Where one of you has special skill in office administration or business management, you can relieve the others of that job. In turn, the other physicians can spend their energies improving patient management skills through attendance at scientific seminars and other activities.

The pooling of funds in the group will allow you to buy more desirable office space, equipment and talents of trained personnel which otherwise would be beyond the reach of the solo practitioner.

Another advantage in joint ventures comes with disability agreements. You can continue to operate a practice even when your partner is disabled. Although the load may be heavy for a while neither one of you will see income dip from illness or other temporary incapacity.

Of course, a disadvantage of having more than one person dispensing services is the increased exposure to legal liability. In today's era of seeming overemphasis on medical malpractice, claims may be made against all participants in a group. This is balanced by a form of built-in peer review which reduces the chance of medical mistakes.

A serious foil to joint ventures is the interference of outsiders—your partners' wives in particular. Unless there is general harmony between all parties, bickerings and jealousies will disrupt the practice of medicine.

Commonly, it is expected that practicing with others will cut the cost of individual overhead and result in greater net income. We do not entirely agree with this concept. To efficiently operate any type of adequate medical plant for each M.D. accommodated, there will be the need for more office space and additional personnel.

Yes, there are some minor benefits in sharing expenses such as your requirement for only one photocopying machine, but generally we see a partnership expense ratio equalling the costs of solo practice.

What Are the Secrets of Successful Partners?

Communication between partners is the secret of a successful medical-business relationship. Your professional partnership is like a marriage and, as with domestic divorce, physician partners can find it exceedingly painful if you finally split.

Marriages that break up often are troubled by three main problems: lack of communication, arguments about money, and unsatisfactory sex life. Excluding the third, broken professional partnerships disintegrate for the same reasons. As unhinged partners you will probably see in retrospect that you looked only at the benefits and disregarded the pitfalls. You will have counted the rewards, but not the frustrations. Naturally, varieties of both are found to be part of your relationship, but you may not have prepared for any disappointments at all.

> *Case in Point:* Charles Barrett and Joseph Davis of Miami, Florida had been practicing together as pediatricians for seven years, and their practice had grown considerably. They were ready to take in another partner.
>
> Bill Sedgewick came in as a pediatric associate on a trial basis for a year. It soon became apparent that Sedgewick had a different work philosophy than the established pediatricians. Barrett and Davis were more rapid-fire types, hard workers seeing a great many children but practicing good medicine. Sedgewick had an easier manner; he wanted to practice slower and get to know each of his young patients and their parents. He wasn't so much attuned to the economics of practice life. The older pediatricians just didn't have the same objectives as the newer man.
>
> This led to a divorce of their potential partnership in a friendly manner. They sat together in conference one day and talked out their differences, which were not reconcilable. Sedgewick walked away from Barrett's and Davis' practice with enough severance pay to keep him going until he set himself up in another practice.

If you wish to form a successful partnership, you have to recognize the true value of discussing the circumstances of practice both in medical and in business aspects. We believe this discussion should be a routine part of your daily practice life. Definitely schedule at least one positive session per week to discuss the circumstances of your patient care and office policies.

One Partner Becomes the Agent of the Other

Partnership involves much more than two or more physicians agreeing to share their profits and losses in an unincorporated business. Legally, each partner is an agent of the other and can bind him by his acts, including contracts, negligence and various commitments. According to a predetermined ratio, they promise to pool capital and labor, share patients and split practice income and expenses between them. But it goes even deeper than that, for once a partnership is decided upon, it becomes absolutely necessary to formalize the association in a document.

Ten Vital Articles to Include in Your Partnership Agreement

Your agreement must describe the terms of the partnership. It should spell out in great detail how the expenses are to be shared and how the income is to be divided.

1. Your document should list the terms of withdrawal—from being established for an indefinite period, to cancellation by either party upon a sixty-day written notice to the other.

Your notice should not be effective in the case of disability of a partner unless the disability continues beyond a six-month period.

2. Income to the partnership will derive from compensation received by any of you from professional sources whether it comes from salaries, patients, hospitals, teaching, publications or any other sale of professional knowledge. Thus, there can be no feeling of displacement of time or publicity that will take away from the practice to accommodate such outside activities.

3. Normally, all operational expenses necessary for the partnership should be included, but there may be special exclusions such as automobile purchase or operation, conventions, books and journals, dues to professional societies, professional entertaining or charitable contributions. By indicating the exclusions, you will eliminate the problems of competition or unfair comparisons.

For example, one of you may have a great deal of professional entertainment expense while the other may be content to not become heavily involved in entertainment for purposes of practice. Such activities may be deductible business expenses for the doctor making the expenditure, but the expenses may not be incorporated in the partnership books.

4. Division of income will best be made on a monthly basis by dividing what is available from the prior month. This distribution would be made on the successive fifteenth of the month.

5. Predetermine accounts receivable, furniture, fixtures, and equipment and any good will as to disposition in the event of the demise or withdrawal of one of you.

It is fairest to figure accounts receivable at 90 percent of the total allowing for the cost of collection and bad debt; or, to acknowledge equities in accounts receivable, the collection ratio as experienced over the last partnership year would be used in the distribution of these funds. The remaining partner should pay over one or two years in twelve or twenty-four payments. This will prevent immediate hardship of paying off too quickly and allow the remaining partner to find professional assistance to replace the withdrawn or deceased partner.

6. Evaluate various capital items at the current market value and get paid over a time period. Good will can be expressed in dollars on the basis of a prior twelve-month period. For instance, you can spell out good will as worth 25 percent of a prior twelve-month net income of the doctor who is leaving.

In a new partnership where the newest member has just entered into practice the 25 percent factor may be used as one-twelfth of a prior twelve months and may graduate each year by one-twelfth until the 25 percent amount is reached. Thus, the second year the newer departing practitioner would receive two-twelfths and the third year three-twelfths which is the maximum 25 percent factor for good will.

7. A disabled partner should not lose his income entirely. Defined disability occurs when your partner cannot discharge his normal duties for more than twenty hours a week. In that instance, he should be entitled to certain compensation during the period of disability according to the following formula:

100 percent of his partnership position for three months; 75 percent for the next three months; 50 percent for the third three months; 25 percent for the final three months; after which we suggest the partnership be dissolved.

8. For time away from practice to attend medical meetings and vacations, equal time for both of you is indicated even though the partnership percentage distribution may not be at parity.

9. Resolve disputes between you by arbitration following the rules of the American Board of Arbitration. For example, within one week after the failure to reach a unanimous decision, each of you should choose an arbitrator who, in turn, will choose a third arbitrator within one week. The three arbitrators listen to the dispute and arrive at a decision by majority vote within a two-week period. The arbitration decision is then made in writing and signed by the arbitrators and mailed separately to each of you. Their decision should be final and binding to all parties and the cost should be a partnership expense.

10. In the event of a voluntary dissolution of the partnership, have the agreement specify exactly what is to happen to the partnership's equipment, telephone number, business records, medical records, and how the retaining partner should compensate the departing partner for these items.

The primary benefits should be granted to the originating physician. In other words, the telephone number should be granted to the physician who really was the solo practitioner and brought in an associate.

JOINING A MEDICAL GROUP

You may prefer to be part of a medical group—"a groupie!"

Medical groups do have tangible professional advantages. One of them is removing some of the economic barriers to acquiring sophisticated equipment. Certainly, the larger the group, the more numerous are its services. You are likely to have more free time and experience a greater variety of patient care.

What Is a Medical Group?

The American Association of Medical Clinics defines a medical group as "Any group of seven or more full-time physicians maintaining a private organization for the purpose of providing general medical care of high quality. Such groups or clinics shall have on their full-time staff at least five physicians in different major specialties, two of which specialties shall be internal medicine and general surgery."

The Council on Medical Service of the American Medical Association defines *group practice* as: "The application of medical service by three or more physicians formally organized to provide medical care, consultation, diagnosis or treatment, through the joint use of equipment and personnel and with income from medical practice distributed in accordance with methods previously determined by members of the group."

The Medical Group Management Association offers yet a third, simpler definition of group practice than the other two: "An organized medical group of three or more doctors of medicine, with common facilities, actively engaged in the practice of medicine and which shall employ a person or persons in the active supervision of its business affairs."

Case in Point: Probably the most highly touted group practice—grown to include several hundred physicians—is the Mayo Clinic. It had its beginning in 1883 when Charles Mayo was joined by his son in the practice of medicine. In seven years the group grew to eight staff members with predominant emphasis on surgery. That was changed later by the addition of a physician who introduced laboratory and X-ray services which formed the nucleus of the medical department.

Types of Medical Groups

With an estimated 38 percent of practicing physicians participating in medical groups, the group practice system seems to be bringing marketplace incentives to the health care industry by making it worth the physician's while to keep his patients as healthy as possible. When they get sick, the group practitioner selects the most efficient and economical methods of care.

Paul M. Ellwood, a Minneapolis physician turned health policy planner, oversees the Health Services Research Center, an arm of the American Rehabilitation Foundation, of which he is president. Dr. Ellwood says, "Only the physician can eliminate unneeded expense. He cannot be policed to do so but must be motivated by professional ethics and organization arrangements that align his economic incentives with those of the consumer. He gets paid [in group practice] for devoting attention to patient education and to disease prevention. He is able to treat his patient in settings that are best for the patient rather than those compromised by what an insurance policy will pay for. He has freer use of allied health personnel."

There are three types of groups in modern medical structuring. One group is comprised of the single specialty; a second consists of multispecialties; the third involves general practice.

The single-specialty group accounts for about half of all groupings. Here, a specialist joins with fellow specialists to work in a joint venture in the incorporated or nonincorporated form. Anesthesiologists, pathologists, radiologists and other hospital-based physicians lend themselves to this form of specialty group. Sometimes pediatricians, orthopedic surgeons, obstetrician-gynecologists, and general surgeons group together as well.

The multispecialty group is composed of three or more physicians practicing in at least two or more fields. One field included will be internal medicine or general practice or general surgery. This group can provide a wider spectrum of medical care with specialists treating specific illnesses in the context of one's total medical care.

The general practice group also provides a wide range of medical care within the confines of family practice. It consists solely of general physicians.

Group Practice Benefits for Patients

The patient gets certain benefits from belonging to the group. They are:

1. The availability of various specialists and technical services at one location.

2. A better assurance of emergency service when needed because of planned full-time coverage.

3. The accumulation of the patient's complete medical history in one file.

4. Access to trained administrative personnel in handling insurance problems or financial difficulties.

5. The patient will benefit, as well, from a built-in peer review. Dr. John P. Bunker, professor of anesthesia at the Stanford University School of Medicine says, "Doctors organized in group practice, where their income depends on the quality of care offered by the entire group, can and do police each other's work."

6. The patient gets more medical practice and better health science for his money because one doctor alone cannot keep up with the rapid advances in medicine today. Internist Ernst R. Jaffe, dean of New York City's Albert Einstein College of Medicine says, "Medicine has become so complex that it's extremely difficult for an individual to be really expert in anything more than a small area. I think we're going to have very few solo practitioners who can live up to the standards that patients and the community have come to expect."

Ten Group Practice Advantages for Physicians

Proponents of group practice health care point out benefits for physicians who participate in one of the group types:

• First, keeping patients healthy is preferable to crisis diagnosis and treatment.

• Second, the health care industry's resources are greater than any patient acting on his own behalf can secure and any physician acting from his office can provide.

In addition, *the ten specific advantages to the physician* of participating in the group practice are:

1. A regular work week with dependable opportunities for leisure.

2. Assurance that your patients are cared for when you attend professional meetings, educational courses, and vacations.

3. Greater accessibility of technical aides and facilities.

4. Ease of consultation.

5. Tending to purely professional problems without concern for administrative matters.

6. The professional stimulus of group relationships in maintaining high quality and improving performance.

7. A sense of professional and economic security through a check on error and full support in adversity.

8. A lower professional and financial investment and more stable income upon entering practice.
9. The availability of the best equipment.
10. The elimination of the direct monetary relationship between doctor and patient, and the presence of competent business management.

Ten Group Practice Disadvantages for Physicians

Of course, group practice holds disadvantages for the physician too. In summary, these are:

1. "Outside" physicians may be reluctant to refer a patient to a specialist member of a multispecialty group for consultation.
2. High-earning specialists usually share some of their earnings with lower-earning partners and realize less income than they would in solo practice.
3. Each group menber shares in the errors of his associates.
4. Each group member must curb his individualistic expression to some degree.
5. Each group member may find himself committed to group decisions of which he disapproves.
6. Each group member may be subjected to restraint of his own expenditures or participate in expenditures of no benefit to him.
7. Undesirable degrees of overspecialization may evolve within the group.
8. Physicians may be attracted to the group who are more interested in professional and personal security rather than in excellence of medical practice.
9. Disagreement over the division of professional income from group service may develop among members.
10. Group members may experience temperamental, interpersonal friction between one another.

Is There an HMO in Your Future?

The prepayment type of group, the *Health Maintenance Organization* or HMO, assures one class of care without respect to age, sex, ethnic or economic group, place of residence or other factor—in the ideal sense. The HMO serves an enrolled population consisting of individuals (or groups of individuals) who contract with it for the range of health services it makes available. The enrolled population is made up of individuals or families in the geographic area who have made a conscious choice, and have entered into a contract with HMO by agreeing to pay (or have paid on their behalf) a predetermined, fixed sum in return for having the HMO assume responsibility for providing the agreed-upon set of health services. A few different types of HMOs exist.

The target area HMO is involved with the population within a health planning area or in a neighborhood health center program. Generally, a target population, although also defined on a geographic base, has made no agreement, either financially or otherwise, to use the services of the center of the planning area.

The enrollment concept differs considerably from the registered population approach that is used by many hospital clinics or health department clinics, as well as by private physicians.

The registered population is one of potential or eligible users of services, who may use the clinic or office for a single service or for many services.

Testimony before the Health Subcommittee of the U.S. Senate Committee on Labor and Public Welfare, on July 20, 1971, indicated that the entire population of the country can be covered either under the plans proposed or the programs now in existence. The enrollee knows the service is there as needed. The HMO knows it is responsible for the enrollee and includes him in its population at risk. The enrollee knows that the agreed-upon services will be paid for if they are obtained from the HMO and not paid for if they are obtained from non-HMO sources.

Using the Kaiser Permanente experience, patients would have medical center facilities: a hospital and ambulatory clinical center where all services are available and are coordinated with neighborhood primary-care clinics situated in peripheral areas. All facilities use a single medical record, and all administrative services are unified. Today this is called "regional planning"; forty years ago it was called "integration and convenience of services for the members."

Patient Care in an HMO

Each personal physician in the HMO group relates to others in a team function. The patient values his relationship with you as his personal physician and relies on you, as does any patient. However, your patient understands at once that there is great value in the unit medical record and that all his radiographs and laboratory findings, from whatever specialist, are all recorded on the same chart, whether he has been an outpatient or bed patient.

HMO services are available to the patient 24 hours a day thanks to the team concept. He knows that if he requires service in the middle of the night and you are not at hand, the unit medical record will serve as a relevant background by which to judge the new emergency. Here is easy access, comprehensiveness, and continuity. The patient does not have to search for it because it is there already.

A population of 25,000 people being served by a health maintenance organization which employs ten to twelve family health teams, is backed up by two pediatricians, two internists, an obstetrician-gynecologist, a general surgeon, a psychiatrist, a nutritionist, a health educator, a social worker and two nurse-midwives. This group of health workers can give comprehensive care, yet function well with a minimum of high cost professionals.

Assuring Effective Utilization of Institutional Facilities

A more highly organized and committed HMO model probably has multi-specialty physicians and other health manpower organized into a *closed-panel group practice*. It uses health facilities owned and operated by the HMO itself. In such an instance, both the group practice and the HMO are devoted to serving the enrolled population groups on a full-time basis with minimal, if any, fee-for-service practice. This model is most closely identified with the Kaiser Foundation Health Plans and the Group Health Cooperative of Puget Sound.

Lesser degrees of organization and structure are represented by HMOs which use either full- or part-time *physician group practices* but have arrangements for *purchase of inpatient care* from community health care facilities. The Health Insurance Plan of New York and the Group Health Association of Washington, D.C. represent this type of organization.

The least degree of organization is represented by HMOs utilizing *individually practicing physicians* and *community health facilities*, bound together by *contractual and professional agreements* and possibly serving the enrolled population side by side with a fee-for-service practice. The Medical Care Foundation Model is exemplified by the San Joaquin Foundation.

In summary: An HMO is a fiscally responsible organization which delivers a full spectrum of health services to a specifically identified and voluntarily enrolled group of persons in return for fixed, prepaid amounts.

Quality of Medical Care in the HMO

Without the fee system's direct financial incentive to hard work how would you assure a continuous high quality of medical care? Would you be sympathetic to the patient's need and feel concern? The answer, a distillation from HMO experience to this point, reveals that quality of care is assured, as in any organization, by a framework of authority and responsibility, backed up by continuous education.

You and other physicians install a safeguard system. You provide surveillance and reasonable professional controls with rewards and penalties as necessary. In any health care system there should be incentives to excellence in the form of both honor and material rewards.

Also, advisory boards of citizens which are made up of both consumers and service providers exercise continuous influence on the appointments of personnel and the operations of the whole health care program. "Consumer control" is replaced by a reasonable mix of consumer-professional collaboration in policy decisions.

REFERENCE FOR CHAPTER FIVE

1. Abrams, William. "Industry beckons M.D.s." *The New York Times,* Nov. 28, 1976.

chapter six

Net More of Your $250,000 Annual Gross This Doctor-Proven Way

I wanted to focus some public attention on the country's forgotten man—the corporation executive paid around $20,000 a year. After taxes and educating his children and perhaps one major illness, he reaches the age of 55 without saving a penny. There's something wrong with the system when a man who does everything he should do ends up in that spot.

— John Ekblom, *New York Herald Tribune,* June 26, 1959.

You can keep more of your annual $250,000 earnings by being the doctor and the corporation rolled into one. Creating a professional corporation pays off with fringe benefits and dividends in the fight to beat inflation.

A corporation is a business entity which permits advantages not available under a partnership or solo proprietorship. It is a legal contrivance formed under the states' enabling acts and possesses articles of incorporation with a board of directors to manage its business. Permitting the establishment of professional corporations has been a boon to practicing physicians.

WHY CONSIDER INCORPORATING AT ALL?

Perhaps the main reason that you would consider incorporation of your practice is that you acquire the advantage of deferred compensations more commonly known as *retirement programs.* Forced saving toward pension fund accumulation is the major attraction. If this is not one of your wants or needs, formation of a professional corporation may not be desirable for you, but it is for most physicians.

Unlike the general nonmedical field however, incorporating does not allow physicians limited liability in the professional corporate form. Also, industry has another advantage of incorporation—flexibility in financing—since a corporation can float a debenture for securing working capital. The doctor who is incorporated cannot do the same.

But there is continuity of practice existence through formation of the corporation, and this is of value. Where two doctors practice together and one leaves the practice, a corporation does not have to be dissolved. Yet, other relative costs for this advantage may be too great and additional aspects of joint practice have to be considered.

Under Section 301.7701-3(b) of the Treasury Regulations, an organization that qualifies as a limited partnership under state law may be classified for purposes of the Internal Revenue Code as an ordinary partnership or as an association taxable as a corporation. It will be treated as an association taxable as a corporation if, applying certain principles set forth below, the limited partnership more nearly resembles a corporation than an ordinary partnership.

The regulations specify six major characteristics ordinarily found in a pure corporation that, taken together, distinguish it from other corporations. These are:

(a) Associates;

(b) An objective to carry on business and divide the gains therefrom;

(c) Continuity of life;

(d) Centralization of management;

(e) Liability for corporate debts limited to corporate property; and

(f) Free transferability of interests.

Whether a particular organization is to be classified as an association taxable as a corporation must be determined by taking into account the presence or absence of these corporate characteristics.

THE ESTABLISHMENT OF ERISA

September 2, 1974 was the day President Ford signed into law the *Employee Retirement Income Security Act* (ERISA), commonly known as the Pension Reform Act of 1974. It is referred to privately by management counselors as "*Every Ridiculous Idea Since Adam.*" ERISA is the most comprehensive, involved and complex statute ever enacted dealing with private pension and profit-sharing plans. Its provisions affect numerous aspects in the design, cost and administration of every qualified plan in existence at the time and those which subsequently have been or will be adopted.

ERISA does the following:

- It effectively taxes at 50 percent any lump sums withdrawn from the average retirement program.
- It encourages an annuity withdrawal that would escape the upper tax rates.
- It makes more stringent fiduciary responsibilities.
- It tightens eligibility standards required for pension and profit-sharing plans.

THERE ARE MANY ADVANTAGES OF AN INCORPORATED PRACTICE

For you, the benefits available as an incorporator begin with employee retirement plans that you may elect to adopt. Such plans offer the use of pretax dollars to accumulate large sums of money for retirement purposes through their deposit by the corporation. The deposits are taken as tax deductions. Thus, assuming your income is taxed at 50 percent, the U.S. Government is, in effect, paying for half of the contribution.

Once deposited in your retirement trust, the funds can be invested in much the same manner as those of any prudent person. Earnings from the investment are tax-deferred and investment decisions can therefore be made without concern for the capital gain holding period. Short-term capital gains, dividends and interest become just as desirable as long-term capital gains.

Limitations on the amounts that can be contributed by your corporation for each employee vary with the type of pension or profit-sharing plan that is adopted. In most cases you may assume that the corporation can contribute an aggregate up to 25 percent of an employee's salary to a combination pension and profit-sharing plan. In some instances the amount allowed can be even greater.

Reimbursed Medical Expenses

Another advantage of incorporation is the medical expense reimbursement. Your corporation can pay all or part of the medical, dental, drug and other related health expenses of your employees and their dependents. You are an employee also. The payments are entirely deductible by the corporation and not taxed as income to you or other employees. Consequently, the 3 percent limitation on the deduction of medical expenses is circumvented on each taxpayer's annual tax return. Within flexible limits it is possible for your corporation to pay more of the medical expenses of its higher salaried employees than of the lower salaried personnel. However, recent legislation has made this area more restrictive. Check with your advisors to assure compliance.

Health insurance premiums, such as for Blue Cross and Blue Shield as well as disability insurance premiums, are considered medical expenses. Before this, most professional people were deprived of any medical expense benefit because the deductible 3 percent of their income was usually much greater than their medical expenses. That is changed with your participation in a professional service corporation.

Deferred Compensation Benefits

We can see immediate benefits from this deferred compensation to retirement years. Deferred compensation is useful for two purposes. It can be applied as a tax-saving device in high income years, thus reducing salary. It could effectively shift income into low income years when the recipient is paying lower taxes.

Consultantship After Retirement

Additionally, your corporation can agree to retain its employees as consultants after their retirement. The retired employees receive reduced salaries, but they must perform only minimal services in order to be entitled to receive payments.

A consultant's agreement can also be used for younger corporate shareholders to repay older shareholders for having taken them into the business without requiring a significant investment. Such situations occur often.

Group Life Insurance

Your professional corporation may purchase up to $50,000 of group term life insurance for each of its employees. The premiums are fully deductible by the corporation and are not taxable to the employee. It is not necessary to buy the same coverage for all employees.

Furthermore, a corporation can pay up to $5,000 to the spouse or other designated beneficiary of a deceased employee. The amount paid is deductible by the corporation and is tax-free to the recipient.

There is greater insulation against liability for others in the corporation.

Taxation Exclusion

Corporate funds not placed in a retirement plan but invested in dividend-yielding stocks are entitled to the 85 percent exclusion from taxation that all corporations enjoy for dividends received.

Common Questions and Answers Concerning Medical Incorporation

Question: *How could a profit-sharing and or pension fund add substantially to my financial position?*

Answer: Monies deposited in such a plan are placed in trust by your professional corporation. The corporation then claims a deduction on its tax return for the amount contributed. There is no tax on the amount deposited as there would have been had you received the money as ordinary income. Once deposited in a trust the funds can be invested in much the same manner as those of any prudent person. Earnings from such invested money in trust are not taxable.

This gives you substantial advantage for short-term gains, dividends and interest. These monies become just as desirable as long-term capital gains. Therefore, you retain funds which might otherwise be lost in taxes and in a manner which dramatically improves your net worth. We have here the advantage of geometric progression. The earnings on the monies which did not go for taxes continue to generate a return until they ultimately become part of a taxable event at the time of their withdrawal.

Question: *Does such a profit-sharing and pension fund permit greater latitude for me in choosing investments?*

Answer: Yes. Because you have a nontaxable fund at your disposal, it may be your decision occasionally to choose a high yield investment in which you have faith. For example, you may believe that a particular company would return 25 percent to the fund. If such a return were in the form of ordinary income, as would be the case in a personal investment, such a venture might *not* be worth considering. On the other hand, because such a return would be nontaxable to the fund, such an investment might be extremely rewarding.

Question: *Will the funds in the pension and profit-sharing fund be available to me at any time?*

Answer: Yes, with certain provisions. You may borrow from a nonintegrated fund under limitations, at just about any time. However, the loan must be collateralized and at current interest rates with a formalized repayment provision.

Question: *How does the profit-sharing and pension fund finally distribute its assets?*

Answer: Upon retirement, you, or any employee, may take a distribution in lump sum with a ten-year forward averaging tax application. In some cases this would not be the most desirable withdrawal. A better arrangement could be for you to choose to withdraw funds under an annuity, incurring ordinary tax rates in the year of withdrawal. Moreover, if you die before taking your distribution in whole or in part, your share of the fund could pass, free of estate tax, to your heirs.

Question: *May I invest the profit-sharing and retirement fund as I please?*

Answer: Yes. With certain prudent guidelines, you have full latitude, but it is wise to seek outside counsel when you make such investment decisions.

Question: *Could the corporation purchase life insurance for me or other employees?*

Answer: Yes. The corporation could purchase up to $50,000 of group term life insurance for its employees. Premiums are fully deductible by the corporation and are not taxable to the individual employee. Additionally, the retirement plan may purchase life insurance with little or no tax significance.

Question: *Could the corporate setup help me to stabilize my income between good and leaner years?*

Answer: Yes. The corporation arrangement permits great flexibility in the displacement of earnings inflow. Because you become a salaried employee of the corporation, a more even and stable flow of take-home pay can result. Such planning may mean additional tax savings since it may be possible to shift income into years when you normally would be in the lower tax bracket. If desired, the corporation may continue to retain you as a consultant after your retirement. You would have to perform only minimal services to be considered such. Then the consultant agreement can be used as a means of payment when the practice is taken on by a younger man who is normally in no position to make a substantial investment.

WHAT DOES FORMATION OF A PROFESSIONAL CORPORATION COST?

Perhaps the most important circumstance involved in considering whether or not you should incorporate your practice is an analysis of the whole cost to do so. Sometimes, unfortunately, the advisor who recommends to a physician that he should incorporate has a personal interest in the decision. There is conflict of interest and as a consequence, many of the costs of incorporating are not delineated.

The following is a list of possible costs incurred when forming a professional corporation:

1. *The employee deferred compensation contribution.* To take advantage of the tax deferral contribution for yourself, you must contribute a like amount or like per-

centage to a pension plan or profit-sharing plan for your employees. What this total expenditure amounts to each year depends upon the number of employees and how much they earn. It could be the means of rewarding and retaining really excellent employees, however.

2. *Employee medical expense reimbursements.* Premium payment for health insurance and other deductible medical expense benefits are collected by the employees along with you. The health insurance plan you institute determines the full premium you will pay for everybody. Of course, this is a highly desirable fringe benefit that you can offer good employees. That way, you are competing with industry for better personnel.

3. *Extra payroll costs because of your employeeship.* As we have mentioned, you become an employee of your corporation, and there are extra payroll costs connected with this status. Social Security costs are higher because both you, as an employee, and the corporation, as your employer, must make contributions to the Social Security Administration. Contributions are made individually to the state unemployment compensation and federal unemployment compensation agencies. There are additional costs to be paid for workmen's compensation.

4. *Accountancy fees and attorney's fees.* Currently, legal origination costs will be about $2,000 with annual legal fees running about $300. Accounting fees are generally about $500 a year higher than for noncorporate practices. Your professional service corporation will be hit with capital stock taxes in some states, franchise taxes, filing fees, corporate income tax requirements, plan administration costs and other costs amounting to approximately $4,000 when everything is totalled. If you pass this first test of feasibility, meeting these operating costs, you will then be forced to answer certain questions in the affirmative prior to establishing your corporation.

We advise *against* forming a corporation if you anticipate higher expenses in the immediate future such as college costs for children that you are not prepared to meet in advance.

We advise *against* incorporation if you cannot get competent legal advice and lack an accountant's help in forecasting and planning corporate financial problems.

We advise *against* incorporating your practice if you cannot live within the rigid rules required of a corporate structure.

The corporation is a separate entity and not a source of paying your personal bills or recklessly paying you bonuses or taking other independent actions. You must hold annual meetings, prepare minutes and document every step of your business life just as do other corporations.

RECOMMENDED CHANGES IN OFFICE PROCEDURE AND MANAGEMENT FOR YOUR NEW PROFESSIONAL SERVICE CORPORATION

1. The telephone numbers for the corporation (which shall be the same numbers which you now have) should be reflected in the *white* pages of every di-

rectory in which these numbers are presently listed. This can be accomplished by having your secretary call your local telephone company business representative. They will make the necessary arrangements to reflect the corporate name and change the billing to the corporate name.

2. The name of the corporation should be added to all appropriate signs and directories in your building.

3. Insurance policies such as office liability, comprehensive, floater and fire and theft should be revised to indicate the existence of the new ownership of the policies. In addition, you should add a "non-owned and lease endorsement" in favor of the corporation to each doctor's automobile insurance policy. Your insurance agent should be able to handle these changes for you. Presently, your malpractice insurance will cover only you and your unincorporated entity. After your corporation is formed, these policies should be endorsed to cover the new corporation.

4. If you are receiving any payments from the department of public aid or the county department of welfare, the corporation's name should be reflected on their records. These agencies will appropriately modify their records if you will write or stamp the corporation's name where your AMA number appears on future consultation reports.

5. Calling cards should be printed with the name of the professional corporation, as well as the individual doctor-employee.

6. Stationery and other printed materials should be printed with the name of the professional corporation, including prescription forms, physical examination reports, surgeon's reports, short forms and final medical reports and forms for insurance company requests for examination and treatment.

7. All accounting records should be kept in the name of the professional corporation, including the accounting records relating to patients and statements issued to them.

8. All purchase-order forms should be printed with the name of the corporation, and suppliers should be notified to bill the corporation and not the individual doctor involved.

9. The professional corporation should maintain a bank account bearing the name of the corporation which will issue all checks in connection with the corporation's affairs. All checks received by the professional corporation for professional services performed by the doctor are to be deposited in this corporate bank account. No fees are to be received or retained by the individual doctor.

10. If leased premises are currently used, the lease should be transferred to the corporation. Your landlord should be able to handle the mechanics of the transfer.

11. All equipment previously leased by the partnership or individual doctor should be transferred to the corporation. The companies who are leasing this equipment should be notified to prepare the proper documents for transfer.

12. The corporation's professional license should be displayed in the corporation's principal office.

13. The corporation should file annual income tax returns and quarterly

federal and state employer tax returns for all employees, including doctor-employees.

14. The corporation should file annual reports with the state when requested, and pay its annual franchise tax on time.

15. When possible, all borrowing from commercial banks should be in the name of the corporation, without individual endorsement or guarantee.

SELF-EMPLOYED (KEOGH) PLANS

The Economic Recovery Act of 1981 contains provisions under which self-employed individuals are permitted to make deductible contributions to their Keogh plans in amounts up to the lesser of 15 percent of net earnings from self-employment income or $15,000 per year, as a maximum. No more than $200,000 of compensation may be taken into account in determining the percentage contributions that would be made from other plan participants. However, if annual compensation in excess of $100,000 is taken into account under the plan, the rate of employer contributions for any participant cannot be less than 7½ percent of that participant's compensation. Contributions may equal 100 percent of earned income up to $750 per year.

Self-employed (Keogh) plans may enter into defined benefit programs (a program that states the retirement benefits to be received and gears the contributions to produce the benefits) for annual earned income up to $50,000 which could increase the contribution beyond the $7,500 level. Such plans can be integrated with Social Security. Much the same as corporate contributions, these self-employed contributions are deductible in a tax year if made before the deadline for filing such tax returns, including extensions.

Moreover, in years during which employees other than owner-employees are covered, an owner-employee may voluntarily contribute, as an employee, up to the lesser of $2,500 or 10 percent of earned income as permitted for employee contributions by common law employees.

THE CORPORATE RETIREMENT PROGRAM COMPARED TO A KEOGH PROGRAM

A. Participation.
   Keogh Plan: A Keogh Plan must cover *all* employees *who have three years of service* (IRS§ 401 (d) (3)).
   Corporate Plan: A corporate plan is required to include a nondiscriminatory cross section of employees who have attained age twenty-five with one year of service (or if plan provides for full immediate vesting, age twenty-five with three years of service) (IRS § 401 (a) (4) and 410 (b).

B. Vesting.
   Keogh Plan: Benefits under Keogh Plan must be *immediately fully vested* (IRS § 401 (d) (2) (A).

Corporate Plan: Corporate plans may provide for deferred vesting (IRS § 401 (a) (7) and 411). Note also, the Conference Committee Report direction to the Internal Revenue Service that, except in cases where intentional discrimination has actually occurred, the Internal Revenue Service accepts a vesting schedule that is not less favorable than the following:

Years of Service	Vested Percentage
Less than 4 years	0
4 years	40
5 years	45
6 years	50
7 years	60
8 years	70
9 years	80
10 years	90
11 years	100

C. Contributions and Benefits
   1. Defined contribution plans.
      Keogh Plan: Keogh *defined contributions plans* are restricted to a maximum contribution of the lesser of:
         (i) 15% of compensation, or
         (ii) $15,000.
      No more than $200,000 of participant compensation may be considered for purposes of the Plan.
      Corporate Plans: May make annual additions up to the lesser of:
         (i) 25% of compensation, or
         (ii) Currently $45,000 (adjusted annually with cost of living index) with no limitations on the amount of compensation considered for these purposes.
   2. Defined benefit plans.
      Keogh Plan: Annual benefit accruals under a *Keogh defined benefit plan* are limited to a scheduled maximum percentage of compensation (with no more than $100,000 being considered), which benefit percentage significantly limits retirement benefits.
      Corporate Plan: Corporate Plans are not so limited but aggregate benefits are generally limited to the lesser of:
         (i) 100% of the high three consecutive years average compensation, or
         (ii) Currently $130,000 (adjusted annually with cost of living index) with no limitations upon compensation considered for purposes of the plan.
   3. Contribution and benefit limitations – employer with both a defined contribution plan and a defined benefit plan.
      Keogh Plan: Combination percentage not to exceed 100%.
      Corporate Plan: A combination of plans may be used in a corporate set-

ting. In any case in which a participant is a participant in both a Defined Benefit Plan and a Defined Contribution Plan maintained by the same employer, the sum of the Defined Benefit fraction and the Defined Contribution fraction may not exceed 1.4.

The Defined Benefit fraction is the result reached from the following fraction:

$$\frac{\text{PROJECTED ANNUAL BENEFIT OF THE PARTICIPANT AT THE CLOSE OF THE YEAR}}{\text{PROJECTED ANNUAL BENEFIT OF THE PARTICIPANT IF THE PLAN PROVIDED FOR THE MAXIMUM BENEFITS ALLOWED BY LAW.}}$$

The Defined Contribution fraction is the result reached from the following fraction:

$$\frac{\text{SUM OF ANNUAL ADDITIONS TO PARTICIPANT'S ACCOUNT AS OF CLOSE OF THE YEAR}}{\text{SUM OF THE MAXIMUM AMOUNT OF ANNUAL ADDITIONS WHICH COULD HAVE BEEN MADE}}$$

As you can see, this area is complex and certainly specifics must be reviewed with the assistance of competent advisors.

4. Employee contributions.

   Keogh Plan: In the case of *Keogh plans,* owner-employee contributions are not permitted unless there are nonowner employees who are permitted to make contributions and when permitted are limited to the lesser of:

   (i) 10% of compensation, or
   (ii) $2500.

   Corporate Plan: In case of *corporate plans,* voluntary contributions may be made by anyone up to 10% of compensation with no maximum limitations other than those imposed through the contribution limitations on annual additions.

   (Note that annual additions include, for purposes of limitations or annual contributions, the lesser of the amount by which contributions exceed 6% of compensation, or ½ of voluntary contributions.)

5. Profit-sharing plan contribution carryover from low profit years.

   Keogh Plan: Keogh profit-sharing plans are not permitted to make larger contributions in one year in order to make up for the absence of a contribution in a preceding year.

   Corporate Plan: In the case of a *corporate profit-sharing plan,* to the extent that a contribution was prevented from being made in one year because of insufficient current and accumulated earnings and profits, such contribution can be carried over to subsequent years (subject to contributions and benefits limitations in such subsequent years).

D. Integration of benefits or contributions with Social Security.
   Keogh Plan: Keogh plans are severely restricted as to integration permitting integration only if such integration does not result in more than ⅓ of employer contributions being applied to owner-employees (IRS §401(d)(6)).
   Corporate Plan: No such restriction applies to corporate plans.
   Corporate defined contribution plans may allocate an amount up to 7% of each employee's compensation in excess of Social Security wage base ($29,700 in 1981) without allocating anything to each employee's compensation at or below the Social Security wage base. Furthermore, defined benefit plans are permitted to provided an offset (reduce defined benefit pensions) by 83⅓% of the primary Social Security retirement benefit or to integrate benefits within certain other alternative formulated limitations.

E. Contribution Formula.
   Keogh Plan: Keogh profit sharing plans are required to have a definite contribution formula.
   Corporate Plan: Corporate plans are permitted to determine the amount of contribution, if any, annually.

F. Forfeitures.
   Keogh Plan: Since contributions to Keogh plans are required to be 100% vested, there are no forfeitures.
   Corporate Plan: Corporate plans may allocate forfeitures among all participants.

G. Distributions.
   Keogh Plan: Keogh plan distributions cannot be made to an owner-employee prior to his attaining age 59½.
   Corporate Plan: Corporate plans can make distribution at any time upon separation of service for other specified reasons.
   1. Tax-free rollover contributions.
      Keogh Plan: Self-employed participants (regardless of whether they are owner-employees) can make rollover contributions to *Individual Retirement Account* plans, but cannot make rollover contributions to another qualified plan or from the *Individual Retirement Account* plan into a qualified plan.
      Corporate Plan: Participants in corporate plans can make tax-free rollover contributions into a qualified plan or into an *Individual Retirement Account* plan and from an *Individual Retirement Account* plan into a qualified plan. (Note: The significance of this difference is that distributions from qualified plans are subject to more favorable tax treatment than those from *Individual Retirement Account* plans, and qualify for estate tax exemption and a $5,000 death benefit income tax exclusion.)

CHECKLIST COMPARISON: NO PLAN, KEOGH PLAN, INCORPORATION PLAN
(x – indicates category principally affected)

NO PLAN	KEOGH	INCORPORATION	
		X	1. Corporate Income Taxes – these would balance with ultimate capital gains on retained earnings
		X	2. Medical Expense Reimbursement Plan
			3. Distribution Factors:
	X		a. Commitment of Keogh to age 59½
		X	b. 20 years plus spreads reflects more favorably for corporation
X	X		c. 20 year minus spreads reflect more favorably to "no plan" and Keogh
X	X		4. Tax Shelter Investing–No Plan doctor and Keogh Plan doctor have more income to take advantage of write-offs and capital gains allowances
		X	5. Vesting and Forfeiture schedules
		X	6. Eligibility standards
		X	7. Estate tax exemptions
		X	8. Group term insurance
		X	9. Death benefit exclusion
		X	10. Dividends earned exclusion
		X	11. Carryover contribution benefits
		X	12. Discretionary vs. definite formula contributions
	X	X	13. Defined benefit plans
	X		14. Voluntary contribution allowances
		X	15. Trustee regulations and investment latitudes
X			16. IRA
		X	17. Problems potential with retained earnings
		X	18. Nuisance value connected with corp. formations
	X	X	19. Cash squeeze analysis
	X	X	20. Double taxations
	X	X	21. Forced savings
		X	22. Limited liability

Note: Readers who desire more information on professional incorporation should acquire *Incorporating the Professional Practice*, Second Edition, Ray, Prentice-Hall, Inc.

H. Estate tax exemption (IRS §2039 (c)).
   Keogh Plan: Amounts in the Keogh accounts of a deceased self-employed individual (regardless of whether an owner-employee) are not eligible for exclusion from federal estate taxes.
   Corporate Plan: Amounts in corporate retirement accounts of any participant are eligible for exclusion from federal estate taxes (if beneficiary properly designated).

I. $5,000 death benefit exclusion.
   Keogh Plan: Amounts in retirement accounts of self-employed individuals not subject to $5,000 income tax death benefit exclusion (IRS §101 (b) (3)).
   Corporate Plan: Lump sum distributions from corporate retirement plans are subject to $5,000 income tax death benefit exclusion (IRS §101 (b) (2) (C)).

J. Trustees.
   Keogh Plan: The trustee of a *Keogh plan* must be a bank or other person approved by the Internal Revenue Service, except where insurance annuity contracts are the sole assets of a Keogh plan.

chapter seven

55 Medical Practice Management Action Ideas With High Six-Figure Potential

Management is now where the medical profession was when it decided that working in a drug store was not sufficient training to become a doctor.

—Lawrence Appley, Past President
American Management Association

Management techniques are applicable to a medical practice just as they are to any business.

Medicine isn't a business, but there is business in medicine, even though many physicians prefer not to face up to the practice problems that the business of medicine presents. However, you can easily function as a businessperson as well as a medical scientist and meet the practicalities of practice life.

THE FOUR "Ps" OF IDEAL MEDICAL PRACTICE MANAGEMENT

Managing a medical practice can be enjoyable once you are properly organized. Organization will come about effectively by following the four "Ps" of ideal medical practice management. They include:

1. Attention to your *patient*
2. Consideration of you, the *physician*
3. Regard for your supporting *personnel*
4. Evaluation of your office *procedures*.

The cultural milieu of the twentieth century, especially in these last two decades, has served as a background for the rise and development of professionalism in practice management as well as in the delivery of medical care.

Practice management is the antidote for the "machine age" in medicine where computers and various sophisticated diagnostic and treatment aids have almost removed "humanity" from the medical art.

The patient sometimes considers himself to be regarded merely as a number on a chart and the diagnosis of his illness mainly based on laboratory reports.

The surgeon may not have seen the patient prior to the operation.

Gone are the days when the family doctor placed his ear on the patient's chest to determine the state of health of his heart or that his lung was congested.

How many doctors are left who diagnose from looking at the patient's eyes, lips, the color of his skin and the odor of his perspiration? Seriously, are the patient's general behavior, the expression on his face and his family problems used as important clues in the diagnosis of disease anymore? Not much! This is why you need the four Ps of practice management. They help you bring humanity back into medical practice and make life easier for you in the bargain.

THE FIRST "P" OF PRACTICE MANAGEMENT: YOUR PATIENT

At all costs, avoid the depersonalization of the patient's personality in your office. Your office exists for your patient's health and welfare and not merely as a place to hang your hat.

Among your supporting personnel, the emphasis should be on one major objective: to give complete and courteous SERVICE. A patient will have a feeling of full confidence when it is reinforced by your well-managed office. Then he knows that he is receiving the best benefits of patient medical care.

Your Best Office Telephone Patterns

Patient care begins with traffic flow, and this originates with the telephone. Effective phone contact will follow a pattern in the modern medical office that extends from a patient to you.

Here are how your office patterns should work:

a. Your receptionist answers the telephone's ring, identifies the office using a calm, smooth, accomplished voice, and secures information from the caller such as the name of the person calling. If the matter is urgent, she learns who the call is about and to whom is the call being made. If illness is acute, she finds out the chief complaints, asks what is the affected body area and the ill person's body temperature. She notes when the trouble started and how often it had occurred before. Then the call back telephone number and the address are recorded for your action.

b. Your receptionist keeps a log of calls indicating all the information she acquired by her questioning and has it available for your attention.

c. Without interrupting you during appointment times with others, except in dire emergencies, the receptionist presents the log at the time set for making return calls—a "boiler room" recall time, in a manner of speaking.

d. At that "boiler room" time you will refer to the patient's charts and medical records with the receptionist's memo of the latest problem, while she dials the patient's number.

e. Recalls should be made on an unlisted line designated just for outgoing calls so as not to tie up the regular lines.

f. Your receptionist must not give advice over the telephone. She has a duty to be firm and to suggest that patients come to the office for treatment rather than allow repeated reliance on the telephone for a patient's medical needs. Emergencies should be steered to the hospital for proper immediate attention, since you really cannot handle the extra involvement because of many appointment obligations.

g. You can contract for portable beepers to alert you to phone messages when you are not in the office. At no cost, the telephone company will survey your phone for busy signals, calls unanswered, and the time it takes your staff to answer the rings.

h. Secure the services of a competent answering service for those times when nobody is in your office. Ask the telephone company to monitor incoming calls to your answering service occasionally to find out how long it takes them to answer.

i. One doctor's telephone bill went down $100 a month when he took outside phones out of examining rooms; waiting patients had been using them for personal calls.

j. Another doctor reduced after-hour phone calls from patients by charging a small fee for those calls.

k. Install a pay telephone in your waiting room to keep patients from tying up your lines. Its availability will generally be welcome.

l. An off-premises extension from the hospital switchboard can be installed in your private office. This will speed contact with hospital personnel and cost as little as $5 a month.

m. One doctor who takes few incoming calls gives some patients a code password or number they can mention to the receptionist to get her to put the call through to him immediately.

n. Instruct your aides that if the patient is angry about something, they should hear him out; let him tell his story without interference or argument; this opportunity for "ventilation" will calm him down.

o. Put a notation on the patient's monthly statement when his insurance form has been filed. It will save extra phone inquiries.

p. If you have a caller who won't get off the phone, push down the hang-up button while *you* are talking—he'll blame it on the telephone company.

q. Another way to end a phone call is to use the excuse that you have a long distance call waiting.

r. Use wall phones instead of desk top instruments whenever possible; they release scarce desk space for other purposes.

s. Touch-Tone® telephone dialing takes three seconds, vs. eight seconds for using a rotary dial.

t. An automatic phone answering machine costs $25 to $30 a month when rented from the telephone company and about $200 when purchased outright.

u. Use an automatic dialing device with tape or card memory for commonly made calls. A model with a memory for 250–500 numbers costs $7.50–$9.50 to rent.

Scheduling Your Appointments

Working from a knowledge of just how much time to allocate for specific types of visits, your receptionist should be scheduling appointments that are punctual without causing you haste in the delivery of individual care. The most favored appointment book is the six-day visual or "week-at-a-glance" manual which allows for scheduling ahead quickly and efficiently. Your time is the most valuable resource the office owns, and it must be preserved for optimum production.

More than one doctor has commented that he is able to leave the office on time only by sticking closely to his appointment schedule. He sidesteps prolonged patient visits by scheduling new additional appointments for this kind of individual who requires more time.

A number of doctors agree that chatting with the patients during office hours is their downfall. Cutting nonmedical dialogue to a minimum helps keep them on schedule.

Office Layout and Space

In Chapter One we spoke of examining room size but did not mention the number of rooms. The formula to follow for how many treatment rooms you should have is to make available as many rooms as you have the capacity to comfortably accommodate patients' needs per hour. That is, if you see three or four patients each hour, have three or four examining rooms equipped and ready for use. They should be multipurpose rooms allowing for several types of medical procedures.

Supply each room with an examining table or patient chair, writing surface, examining light, a sink, waste receptacle and provisions for storage of all the usual medical items utilized routinely. Light switches for the room and examining light should be within arm's reach.

The Process of Patient Exit

At no time give your patient his medical record to bring to the receptionist. Rather, issue routing slips that indicate the fee for services rendered and when you want subsequent appointments scheduled. Have the routing slip prenumbered for audit control, and instruct the patient to return this slip to your receptionist. The receptionist's responsibility, in turn, is to solicit payment and to do the rescheduling, if indicated.

Often enough, patient exit time will usually be the moment your patient chooses to tell you of personal and quasi-medical problems. One group practice in Phoenix, Arizona is effectively using a full-time psychologist to consult with patients about these various personal problems that need talking out. Previously it was done by doctors in the group, but the patients now pay a regular fee for this service, and the group reports no patient criticisms.

THE SECOND "P" OF PRACTICE MANAGEMENT: YOU, THE PHYSICIAN

Managing is an all-encompassing concept, and it applies to you, the physician, just as much as it does to other facets of your practice. Poor self-management is generally defined as the failure to put a high enough value on your time. You have to be disciplined.

Besides knowledge, *time* actually is the only thing you sell; yet, time is what you have the least of. The second "P" of practice management might better be labeled "physician time."

A number of doctors report an increase in patient office visits as the result of properly delegating tasks and shifting work loads. The problem in most medical offices today is how to take care of an overabundance of patients. Surely, you don't want to schedule patients who do not require scheduling.

Having the appropriate people perform appropriate tasks makes for a faster, more efficient office routine and gets more of people's needs fulfilled.

The most serious failing an employee can have is to waste your professional and personal time. Make sure your staff knows that. Don't let them reduce your productivity with incorrect scheduling. More effective delegation will automatically increase your productivity and income.

> *Case in Point:* One in-hospital based physician, E. Jones Marks of New Orleans, lost a major portion of his income when he was disciplined for his time delinquency. His hospital administrator finally yielded to the numerous complaints made against the doctor and asked for his resignation from the hospital. This also seriously affected his employability at other institutions as well.

In a survey of physicians on the subject of productivity taken in 1974, Maynard L. Haecox, Program Director of Practice Management, the Division of Medical Practice, American Medical Association, asked:

1. Do you think that you could improve your productivity by 5 percent?
2. If you could improve production, why would you want to?

Some of the answering physicians said they would not change any methods to improve their productivity in order to make more money. Money was the least important thing. One doctor remarked, "The government will simply take it away from me."

The two major reasons physicians gave for wishing to increase productivity were:

A. To have more time for themselves and to spend with their families,
B. To more effectively handle more patients that they must now turn away.

Haecox told us, "The ever-increasing cost of doing business and the public opinion constraint on unlimited fee will undoubtedly level off eventually. As of today, however, these factors are reducing the doctor's profit margin to a point where he may have already decided that the second car in the family does not have to be a Cadillac or a Mercedes Benz."

Thus, increased productivity may not be motivated by the desire for increased income, but rather by the longing for more personal time.

Reading Time Required

A few doctors told us that slow reading habits had hindered their productivity but speed reading techniques enabled them to reduce time spent with correspondence, medical reports, and business and professional journals.*

In the interest of continuing your education, you must establish a workable strategy for more effective reading. We suggest that you set aside at least one half-day per month for just reading.

To determine what to read, follow the advice of some communications experts. They recommend that you systematically examine the contents of your practice—what problems you lean toward as a specialty and see the most of—and focus your efforts on that kind of clinical reading. Then again, read material on subjects you feel the least confident about. Once you make this evaluation, seek out those kinds of matters and develop a reading list in those particular subjects.

Another good suggestion is to catch up on reading what you have set aside by isolating yourself for a full weekend at an out-of-the-way place. Just remain totally on your own to study literature and think through the prior month's activities. Then plan the next month's activities. That way, you can cover more reading material at a deeper level of concentration and analyze what you have done and what you will do. The obstacle to weekend isolation may be in finding such a time block which won't play havoc with the rest of your schedule.

Thirty-Two Tips for Saving Your Time

This whole area of time management has constantly been a problem for physicians. "Time is life," wrote Alan Lakein.[1] "It is irreversible and irreplaceable. To waste your time is to waste your life, but to master your time is to master your life and make the most of it."

To help you make every minute count we have supplied thirty-two time-saving suggestions many doctors find effective:

---

*A program of accelerated reading is presented in *Breakthrough Rapid Reading*, by Peter Kump. Parker Publishing Company, Inc., West Nyack, N.Y. 10994.

ACTION IDEAS WITH SIX-FIGURE POTENTIAL 117

1. Physicians in group practice have discovered a real time saver for hospital rounds and nursing home visits. On a rotating basis, one practitioner attends all of the group's noncritical patients and reports back to the respective physician responsible.

2. Routine house calls have been eliminated by most general practitioners.

3. GPs have cut out obstetrical work because they feel their time involvement is disproportionately high in this area.

4. Physicians in urban areas have tried admitting their patients into just one hospital, thus avoiding multiple hospital trips.

5. For medical records, some doctors suggest keeping simple, well-organized notes instead of verbose narration. It saves time both in the compilation of the record and in retrieving information from the record.

6. Many doctors have developed an effective telephone screening procedure, thereby avoiding constant interruptions. The procedure elected must be individually determined since each doctor's considerations vary.

7. One physician found that by eliminating hospital corridor consultations with patients and hospital employees he was able to shave off a sizable chunk of time earmarked for hospital rounds.

8. Some M.D.s have worked out systems with their hospital administrators which allow them—whenever possible—to have all their patients located on the same floor or in one section of the hospital.

9. Others find that having direct telephone lines going into central dictation equipment at the hospital is a godsend for clinical record keeping.

10. Many schedule detail men's visits right in with patient appointments. Some physicians combine their coffee breaks with these ten-minute detailing slots. A few have their nurse talk with the detail men and then report any pertinent information to the doctor.

11. One doctor told us that he saves time on hospital rounds and gets his daily exercise by climbing stairs rather than waiting for elevators.

12. The first thing in the morning is when you should set priorities for the day. Plan your schedule. Make a list and tick it off as the important items come up. Start with the most profitable parts of big projects.

13. Give yourself a break with a segregated pocket of time for hobbies and relaxation.

14. Of course, you are almost obligated to fill out health insurance forms for patients, but you may be able to cut down on the inflow of paper, or at least make a little money from the insurance form snowstorm by charging for the execution of additional forms beyond one or two. Doctors do generally charge from $3 to $5 per extra form.

Note that the only real way to eliminate the insurance paperwork is to eliminate the paper. This may be finally accomplished by computers but probably not for several years yet. The Health Insurance Council standard claim form may be the best news in years to eliminate some paperwork.

15. Save time by issuing printed instructions to the pharmacist or the pa-

tient on prescription blanks. Perhaps you could use a checklist that is preprinted. Your nurse can fill in the patient's name and address.

16. Compile standing preadmission orders to a hospital that cover the admitting diagnosis most common in your practice.

17. Educate your patient in advance about the hospital procedures for admission that relate to his condition.

18. Write orders that inform the hospital staff of the patient's situation and special needs and make them a part of the patient's hospital chart.

19. Have your aide pull all scheduled patient records for the day in advance of office operations. Perhaps do it the night before.

20. Take advantage of dictation procedures as much as possible. Write longhand as little as you can. It takes too much time.

21. Use a self-administered history form that your patient can complete before you see him.

22. Short of revealing too much about his condition and treatment, have your aide field the patient's questions beforehand.

23. Ask your aide to perform routine procedures and record measurements such as weight, blood pressure, etc. prior to your entrance into the examining room.

24. Reduce the billing process by requiring your receptionist to tactfully encourage cash payments at the time of visits.

25. Use color coding where feasible for a more total control operation in the office. Color-coded tags on the outside of examining room doors, for instance, will let you and your personnel see at a glance and from a distance what the status of the room is at any given moment.

26. Provide a private space in which your receptionist can discuss the bill and other matters with the patient. It speeds collections and reduces billing costs.

27. Mount less frequently used equipment such as the EKG on a cart to be able to move it from room to room. Don't move the patient if you can avoid it.

28. Set out an area for normal traffic flow patterns. For example, give routine injections in a particular spot out of the way of other activities so as not to interfere with the main office routine.

29. Install chart holders on the outside of examining room walls or on the door, in which your assistant can insert the patient's chart. That way, you can look the chart over before entering the room.

30. Obtain rubber stamps for frequently repeated information such as name and address, common diagnosis, your signature, etc. However, use caution with those rubber stamps, especially the one containing your signature.

31. Establish a standard fee schedule to which your collection aide can adhere. Formulate it from reconciling with the Blue Shield list of fees, a relative value guide, and from consulting with other physicians in your community.

32. If you become caught up in the time-consuming giant called "committee work," you can improve your lot by budgeting time allotments for this work. Then communicate your time budget to all interested parties; stick to this time budget. (See Figure 7–1.)

FIGURE 7–1

AGENDA FOR MEETING

FROM: _____

TO: _____

NAME OF ORGANIZATION: _____

PLACE AND TIME: _____
_____

Time Table	General Subject	Specific Items	Individual Responsible

PLEASE

Be on time as the meeting will start on schedule.
Prepare your remarks in advance of the meeting.
Limit discussions to only those topics outlined in the agenda.

Follow the timetable organizing your presentation for the best utilization of your allotted time.

Avoid long debates with opposing views. Think it out by yourself away from the full committee meeting.
Do not permit interruptions of the meeting by receiving nonemergency calls during the stated meeting hours.

Seven Hints for Extended Periods Out of Your Office

Many physicians continue office operation with full- or part-time staffing when they are away for extended periods of time. Your productivity and income can be maintained in a very effective manner if your office personnel plan their use of time.

Here are seven hints for when you are away:

1. Make a written plan of activities during this time for each staff member.
2. If it is unnecessary to have the entire staff on tap, designate who is to have which time off before you leave.
3. Put someone in charge and make sure everyone knows it.
4. If some clinical activities are to continue, insure that the responsible nurse has appropriate physician coverage and instruction.
5. If there are certain things you do *not* want done, *write* them down and confirm that everyone understands.
6. Give very specific information as to where you will be at all hours while you are away. If there are changes in your plans, call your office to quickly alert the staff.
7. If your staff has done a good job while you were away, reward them, as a group, as soon as possible on your return. A special luncheon, dinner or show is a good idea.

Ten Office Tasks to Be Accomplished While You Are Away

Here are ten possible tasks that can be done while you are out of the office for a time:

1. Do complete and thorough housecleaning.
2. Check and reorder all necessary supplies.
3. Update medical records and other paperwork.
4. Complete all backlogged insurance forms for your signature.
5. Use the telephone for an all-out attempt at collecting overdue balances.
6. Audit and complete any bookkeeping.
7. Catch up on all tickler files, especially periodic and special examinations.
8. Do a front office practice profile.
9. Make hospital visits (by your office nurse) to check on needs of patients who may be under the care of someone covering for you.
10. Repaint the office rooms that require it.

THE THIRD "P" OF PRACTICE MANAGEMENT: SUPPORTING PERSONNEL

Rare is the physician today who does not need at least one extra pair of hands in the form of an office assistant. Perhaps at some past time your success or failure in practice rested on your shoulders alone, but that is no longer the case. You need an assistant who understands the job, improvises where required, works efficiently, respects you, is loyal to you, and shows concern for patients. No matter how many people work for you or what their functions are, those functions should be part of all the employees' particular requirements.

The search for medical office aides is among the most difficult and frustrating undertakings in professional practice. Finding the person most suitable to do a job is like finding a precious stone in a sunken treasure galleon. Consequently, one of the poorest economies is to offer an austere salary program. An investment in good personnel pays the best dividends in the long run.

New employees will be dealing with sick people; this takes skill and tact. You will want them to generate good feelings in your patients. To do this, employees have to feel good about themselves and the conditions under which they work.

The number of capable, educated, fine-quality medical assistants seems to be diminishing steadily. This state of affairs may exist because of three reasons:

- With greater volumes of patients and more sophisticated medical equipment, the demand for skilled assistance has increased.
- Being a member of a modern, multimember hospital or clinic staff offers more advantages than being a single or double member of a doctor's office.
- Industry competes with physicians by offering unbeatable extra pay benefits such as profit-sharing plans, retirement funds, sick leave pay, long vacations, high salaries, attractive job conditions, shorter hours, hospitalization, socializing among employees, and other attractions.

The Hiring Procedure for Supporting Personnel

Supporting personnel in your practice are by definition, or by expectancy, an extension of yourself. They can build or tear down your image to the outside world, to patients in the office, and over the telephone. Projection of your image should be one of cheerfulness, tactfulness, neatness, industriousness, and friendliness. It is up to you to make sure your employees represent you that way, and it all begins with your hiring procedure.

We advise you to recruit applicants with a blind advertisement placed in your local newspaper. For example:

```
CHALLENGING POSITION
In Progressive Professional Office
Awaits
Enthusiastic Person
Who Enjoys
Working With People
Good Starting Salary With
Increases And Individual Growth
Give References And Work History
Contact Box 0000
```

Recruiting this way avoids a parade of unsuitable persons marching through your office and allows for a relaxed scrutiny of applicants. Your first opportunity to appraise individuals will then be through their handwriting or spelling in their answering letters. In response to what is said or how it is written, you may next choose to ask a series of pertinent questions by mail. Mail examinations of this nature are less time-consuming than personal interviews.

Call in the top three candidates for the job you are offering and talk to them yourself. If those three turn out not to be probable choices call in the next three.

Before your interview, give the candidate a report form to fill out in the office. (We illustrate this form in Figure 7–2. Reprints of the "Application for Employment," form #08281, are available from the Amsterdam Printing and Litho Corp., Amsterdam, N.Y. 12010.) You will be able to use the interview report to record your initial personal impressions and later to recall the interview when weeding out applicants.

Naturally there are other good sources from which to recruit job applicants. One of the best is word-of-mouth among colleagues. Then there are selected patients and former employees who may have friends looking for a job. Post a notice on the nurses' bulletin board at your hospital. Contact a good secretarial school or business college and tell them of your requirements for an effective clerical assistant. The state's employment agency is always anxious to receive new job openings as are every medical employment agency and general employment agencies.

If you can personally telephone and invite a candidate to come for the interview, do so. Telephoning will give you a chance to hear his or her phone personality during the first moments of surprise. At the same time you will be able to ask about the facts in the candidate's letter of application.

The office interview is vital, since it is the primary way you have to judge the potential employee's character and personality. Don't be fooled by a person who counts on talking his way into a job while covering up a neurosis or some other internal need to have a doctor sympathize with past or present troubles. Doctors' offices are notorious for attracting this type of applicant.

Immediately after the interview, telephone the candidate's previous employers and ask about the individual's honesty, industry, quick-wittedness and other abilities. The form shown in Figure 7–3, a telephone reference for interviewing the applicant's former employer, is of great value when contacting the applicant's references.

Make a credit check too. If a person cannot pay his bills, he might be tempted to institute some unauthorized profit-sharing from your income. White-collar embezzlement has been a bane of small office employers.

Case in Point: Thomas Rogan, an internist practicing in Cedar Rapids, Iowa, had an office assistant who embezzled him out of an estimated $11,000. His collection system made use of receipts that left a carbon record for the accountant. It was numerically controlled so that the doctor thought he had security. The embezzler would insert a card measured to just the right size be-

FIGURE 7-2

To Applicant: We deeply appreciate your interest in our organization and assure you that we are sincerely interested in your qualifications. A clear understanding of your background and work history will aid us in placing you in the position that best meets your qualifications *and* may assist us in possible future upgrading.

PERSONAL   Date: _____

Name _____ Social Security No. _____
         Last   First Initial   Middle Initial

Present address _____ Telephone No. _____
         No.   Street   City   State   Zip

How long have you lived at above address? _____

Previous address _____ How long did you live there? _____
         No.   Street   City   State   Zip

To Applicant: READ THIS INTRODUCTION CAREFULLY BEFORE ANSWERING ANY QUESTIONS IN THIS BLOCKED-OFF AREA. The Civil Rights Act of 1964 prohibits discrimination in employment practice because of race, color, religion, sex or national origin. P.L. 90-202 prohibits discrimination on the basis of age with respect to individuals who are at least 40 but less than 65 years of age. The laws of some States also prohibit some or all of the above types of discrimination.
 DO NOT ANSWER ANY QUESTION CONTAINED IN THIS BLOCKED-OFF AREA UNLESS THE EMPLOYER HAS CHECKED THE BOX NEXT TO THE QUESTION, thereby indicating that the requested information is needed for a bona fide occupational qualification, national security laws, or other legally permissible reasons.

☐ Are you over the age of twenty-one? _____ If no, hire is subject to verification that you are of minimum legal age.

☐ Sex: M _____ F _____   ☐ Height: _____ ft. _____ in.   ☐ Weight: _____ lbs.

☐ Marital Status: Single _____ Engaged _____ Married _____ Separated _____ Divorced _____ Widowed _____

☐ Date of Marriage _____ ☐ Number of dependents including yourself _____ ☐ Are you a citizen of the U.S.A.? _____

☐ What is your present Selective Service classification? _____

☐ Indicate dates you attended school:

Elementary _____ High School _____ College _____
         From   To   From   To   From   To

Other (Specify type of school) _____
                                         From   To

☐ Have you ever been bonded? _____ If yes, on what jobs? _____

☐ Have you been convicted of a crime in the past ten years, excluding misdemeanors and summary offenses? _____ if yes, describe in full _____

Employer may list other bona fide occupational questions on line below:
☐ _____

What method of transportation will you use to get to work? _____

Position(s) applied for _____ Rate of pay expected $_____ per week

Would you work Full-Time _____ Part-Time _____ Specify days and hours if part-time _____

Were you previously employed by us? _____ If yes, when? _____

List any friends or relatives working for us _____
                                                    Name(s)

If your application is considered favorably, on what date will you be available for work? _____ 19_____

Are there any other experiences, skills, or qualifications which you feel would especially fit you for work with the Company? _____

FIGURE 7–2, continued

Do you have any physical defects which preclude you from performing certain kinds of work? _____ If yes, describe such defects and specific work limitations. _____

Have you had a major illness in the past 5 years? _____ If yes, describe _____

Have you received compensation for injuries? _____ If yes, describe _____

RECORD OF EDUCATION

School	Name and Address of School	Course of Study	Check Last Year Completed	Did You Graduate?	List Diploma or Degree
Elementary			5 6 7 8	☐ Yes ☐ No	
High			1 2 3 4	☐ Yes ☐ No	
College			1 2 3 4	☐ Yes ☐ No	
Other (Specify)			1 2 3 4	☐ Yes ☐ No	

MILITARY SERVICE RECORD

Were you in U.S. Armed Forces? Yes _____ No _____ If yes, what Branch? _____

Dates of duty: From _____ To _____ Rank at discharge _____
                  Month Day Year   Month Day Year

List duties in the Service including special training _____

Have you taken any training under the G.I. Bill of Rights? _____ If yes, what training did you take? _____

PERSONAL REFERENCES (Not Former Employers or Relatives)

Name and Occupation	Address	Phone Number

FIGURE 7-2, continued

List below all present and past employment, beginning with your most recent

	Name and Address of Company and Type of Business	From Mo.	From Yr.	To Mo.	To Yr.	Describe in detail the work you did	Weekly Starting Salary	Weekly Last Salary	Reason for Leaving	Name of Supervisor
I										
II										
III										
IV										
V										

May we contact the employers listed above? _____ If not, indicate by No. which one(s) you do not wish us to contact _____

The facts set forth above in my application for employment are true and complete. I understand that if employed, false statements on this application shall be considered sufficient cause for dismissal. You are hereby authorized to make any investigation of my personal history and financial and credit record through any investigative or credit agencies or bureaus of your choice.

In making this application for employment I also understand that an investigative consumer report may be made whereby information is obtained through personal interviews with my neighbors, friends, or others with whom I am acquainted. This inquiry includes information as to my character, general reputation, personal characteristics and mode of living. I understand that I have the right to make a written request within a reasonable period of time to receive additional, detailed information about the nature and scope of this investigative consumer report.

_____
Signature of Applicant

3

FIGURE 7-2, continued

APPLICANT—Do not write on this page
FOR INTERVIEWER'S USE

INTERVIEWER	DATE	COMMENTS

FOR TEST ADMINISTRATOR'S USE

TESTS ADMINISTERED	DATE	RAW SCORE	RATING	COMMENTS AND INTERPRETATION

REFERENCE CHECK

*Position Number	RESULTS OF REFERENCE CHECK	*Position Number	RESULTS OF REFERENCE CHECK
I		IV	
II		V	
III			

*See Page 3

4

FIGURE 7–3

TELEPHONE REFERENCE CHECKING QUESTIONNAIRE

Applicant's Name _____   Check (✓)
Person Contacted _____ Telephone _____ Question (?)
Position _____

1. **Skills**—How did you find the quality and speed of work in the following areas:
   (1) typing? _____
   (2) dictation? _____
   (3) other? _____

2. **Personality & Attitudes**
   (a) Employment stability   —How long did she work with you? _____
                                 —Why did she leave? _____
   (b) Interest in people   —Did she interrelate well with:
                                    (1) your patients? _____
                                    (2) your staff? _____
   (c) Organizational ability   —Was she well organized _____
   (d) Intelligence   —Did she come up with useful suggestions to improve the office? _____
                                 —Could she solve problems without a lot of interaction with you? _____
   (e) Conscientiousness &   —Was she conscientious? _____
       thoroughness   —Did she complete her work thoroughly? _____
   (f) Initiative & leadership   —Did she create useful projects for herself and complete them? _____
                                 —Would you say she has good leadership capabilities _____
   (g) Maturity   —As situations arose did she handle them with maturity and good judgment? _____
   (h) Positive attitude   —Was she cheerful and enthusiastic about her work and the people around her? _____
   (i) Alertness   —Was she usually attentive and alert? _____

3. **Evaluation**
   (a) Was she punctual? _____
   (b) Did she have good attendance? _____
   (c) What were her main faults? _____
   (d) What was the most significant problem you have had with the person? _____
   (e) Would you rehire her? _____

tween the sheets of the receipt blanks. When the patient paid $50, the embezzler provided a top sheet receipt to the payee with the correct amount. Then she would remove the cardboard to mark $25 in blue pencil on the carbon control page and record $25 onto the final day statement. Then she would put $50 onto the patient payment record.

The doctor didn't catch her for two years because he never went to the patient payment record to compare it with the carbon control page or the final day statement.

Rate the applicant on your interview report form that is part of Exhibit 7–2, the "Application for Employment." Look for that person with the highest number of positive impressions and call back your best candidate. Do not hire a person much below his or her asking price. Instead, anticipate that your new assistant is going to be so superior that he or she will soon advance to the highest salary this individual ever earned because of performance.

Hire with a probationary period of three months. Before starting work, the new employee must be told all the drawbacks of the job such as Saturday work, overtime hours, short lunch periods, lack of fringe benefits, etc. Let there be no surprises!

Request that the new assistant seek help from others on the staff or from you in duties where he/she may be unsure of what is required.

After the probationary period passes and there is proof that the employee has grown steadily in value, make a small salary adjustment upward. A subsequent annual review should net more salary increases based upon performance coupled with the rise in the cost of living. Maintain a personnel file for each person on your staff for your reference.

Maximize Your Assistant's Assistance with an Employee Policy Manual

Medical assistants, new or experienced, need ongoing indoctrination by you—their physician-boss. Spell out standard office procedure in an *employee policy manual* prepared for the whole staff. In it should be job descriptions for each staff position so that no problems arise from job crossovers. Delineate office rules and requisites. Have employees understand about periodic salary reviews, paid vacations, paid holidays, holidays that fall on employee days off, employee appearance, fringe benefits, confidentiality, and anything else you can add that affects your practice. Make sure the manual stays current since it can be the source of information for a new assistant replacing an experienced person who must leave your employ suddenly.

Here are some typical policies you may elect for inclusion in your employee office manual:

• New employees shall receive a salary review at the end of three to six months of employment and thereafter at the end of each twelve-month period of consecutive employment. These reviews will take place for all staff members at the same time at the end of the fiscal or calendar year.

• Part-time employees shall receive the hourly rate and fringe benefits proportionate to full-time employee rates in the same position.

• After three months of employment, the employee may be granted a half-day of paid sick leave for each month of employment up to six working days per year.

• After six months of employment there are five working days of paid vacation granted. After one year of employment there are ten working days of paid vacation; after five years, fifteen working days of paid vacation; after ten years, twenty working days.

• Sick leave or vacation days not consumed during the year would not be looked upon as accruing to overlap into the next year. Rather, there is a bonus arrangement to accommodate for those days not taken off. (This becomes a nice incentive plan.)

• An employee may take a leave of absence for three days without loss of salary for some important occurrence—a death in the family, for instance.

Optional Inclusions in Your Employee Relations

Hold regular office personnel meetings with formal agendas, and interpret the employee policy manual when required. Like it or not, as the physician-boss, you are the health team leader, and you must instill in your assistants the feeling that you value their assistance. To do this in the most effective way, take note of the tips we offer in two subsections that follow this one about employment performance appraisal.

To maximize the assistants' assistance, request that they continue with their medical education. Give them items of professional interest to read. Discuss why you prefer one technique over another and why you treated Mrs. Morris one way and Mrs. Papas another even though they have similar health problems.

Clearly establish starting times and deadlines, delegate responsibilities, maintain job descriptions, and itemize lists of each assistant's duties. The employee policy manual should tell it all, but you should supplement instructions with friendly asides.

Stress the importance of keeping the confidences of patients inside and outside the office. Prevail upon them not to discuss illnesses of people or their personal lives. Even if a patient asks a question about his own case, instruct your assistants to refer that inquiry to you.

Also stress the team approach to maximize your assistants' assistance.

Since the field of health care is one of the most satisfying areas in which an individual can build a career, don't overlook offering a helping hand to one of your assistants if he or she desires to continue with more formal education in the field.

Six Tips for the Pre-Performance Appraisal

Steps to be taken before you do a pre-performance appraisal of your various employees:

1. Hold a performance appraisal conference with every employee, at regular intervals, as a means of maintaining employee morale. Use the performance appraisal conference to also determine directions for future growth in work skills

so as to provide a rational basis for salary review and possible redefinition of job duties.

2. Tell employees of your performance evaluation policy, either at the time they are hired, or at a time well before the day when the first conference takes place.

3. Before the conference you should set aside some time for a solitary, careful study of the employee's job behavior. Carefully check off the box scorings on a form marked for "Employee Performance Appraisal" illustrated in Figure 7–4.

Evaluate the employee's work in specific task areas, preferably with the help of a written job description. Compile a list of personality or behavioral characteristics you believe are important to the job, and rate the employee in these areas. Remember, this is done before you consult with your employee.

FIGURE 7–4

EMPLOYEE PERFORMANCE APPRAISAL _____ ÷ 8 = _____

4.1 TO 5.0	EXCELLENT
3.1 TO 4.0	GOOD
2.6 TO 3.0	FAIR
1.6 TO 2.5	MEDIOCRE
1.0 TO 1.5	UNSATISFACTORY

NAME OF REVIEWER _____

(USE SPACE BELOW FOR ADDED COMMENTS)

_____

DATE DISCUSSED WITH EMPLOYEE _____

EMPLOYEE'S SIGNATURE _____

FIGURE 7–4, continued

PROFESSIONAL ECONOMICS & MANAGEMENT
EMPLOYEE PERFORMANCE APPRAISAL

NAME _____ DATE _____

JOB TITLE _____ SALARY _____

STARTING DATE OF EMPLOYEE _____ DATE OF LAST REVIEW _____

COOPERATION
Does This Employee Show Ability and Willingness To Get Along With Doctors and Co-Workers?

5	4	3	2	1
Exceptional team worker. Flexible.	Usually agreeable. Tactful and obliging.	Goes along willingly.	Sometimes uncooperative.	Tends to cause friction.

DEPENDABILITY
How Reliable Is The Employee In Meeting Work Schedule?

5	4	3	2	1
Places office interests ahead of personal conveniences.	Punctual. Does not waste time.	Generally on the job as needed.	Some abuses. Occasionally needs to be admonished.	Chronic abuses of work schedule.

INITIATIVE
How Well Does This Employee Begin An Assignment Direction and Recognize The Best Way Of Doing It?

5	4	3	2	1
Self starter. Makes practical suggestions.	Proceeds on assigned work voluntarily and readily accepts suggestions.	Does regular work without prompting.	Relies on others. Needs help getting started.	Must usually be told exactly what to do.

JOB KNOWLEDGE
How Well Does This Employee Understand The Job To Which Assigned?

5	4	3	2	1
Thoroughly understands all aspects.	More than adequate knowledge of job.	Has sufficient knowledge to do job.	Insufficient knowledge of some phases.	Continually needs instructions.

LEADERSHIP
Is The Employee Capable Of Supervising Others?

5	4	3	2	1
Exceptional leader and organizer.	Plans work well. Poised, respected.	Has adequate leadership qualities.	Potential leader but needs development.	Poor planner & organizer. Fails to develop and inspire others.

PATIENT AWARENESS
Is The Employee Genuinely Concerned How The Patient Is Made Welcome To The Practice?

5	4	3	2	1
Always shows concern about patient's welfare and comfort.	Usually careful about patient's well being.	Average concern for patient's feelings.	Sometimes short and inconsiderate of patients.	Never regards interest of the patient. Patients have complained about employee.

PERSONAL WORK HABITS
How Accurate, Neat and Complete are the employee's work habits?

5	4	3	2	1
Always neat, accurate and thorough.	Few mistakes. Careful worker.	Work is acceptable.	Occasionally careless. Needs checking.	Inaccurate and careless.

RESPONSIBILITY
How Does This Employee Accept All The Responsibilities of The Job?

5	4	3	2	1
Accept all responsibilities fully and meets emergencies.	Conscientiously tries to fulfill job responsibilities.	Accepts but does not seek responsibility.	Does some assigned tasks reluctantly.	Indifferent. Avoids responsibilities.

4. If you feel the employee's work was unsatisfactory in certain areas, you should try to isolate the possible reasons.

   a. Were the job responsibilities and standards of performance inadequately communicated?
   b. Did the employee misunderstand the relative importance of a particular task as compared to other tasks?
   c. Is the employee's work deficient because of attitudinal problems? Is the employee too heavily involved with personal activities?
   d. Is the employee inadequately trained for the task?
   e. Is the employee sincerely concerned about doing a good job?
   f. What supervisory techniques seem to work best with the employee?

5. Unsatisfactory performance does not automatically call for dismissal but may mean dismissal should be considered. Answers to the questions listed above may suggest measures to remedy the employee's performance.

6. Identify and define areas of performance in which your employee is satisfactory or above the required level. Consider new ways of utilizing the employee's talents. Find some things about which to compliment the person.

Ten Tips for the Actual Performance Appraisal

How to conduct the interview for performance appraisal of one of your staff members:

1. The interview should be conducted in a neutral setting rather than in the work areas normally used by either you or your aide. Make an effort to avoid all interruptions. Perhaps you could take the employee to lunch if you have only good impressions to report. On the other hand, if you suspect that the conference is going to be unpleasant or you may be discharging the person, try to confer in the employee's office so that you can leave the room when you wish.

2. The interview should never be conducted immediately after the employee has made a serious mistake or something went seriously wrong in the office. If necessary, postpone the interview until a later time.

3. At the beginning of the interview, establish an atmosphere of two-way communication. Let the employee know you are interested in his or her viewpoints and will need his or her active help.

4. Make maximum use of the person's satisfactory or superior areas of performance. Mention them both before and after you talk about the unsatisfactory ones.

5. In general, try to concentrate on talking about behavior and facts rather than opinion, beliefs, values, and attitudes.

6. In dealing with an unsatisfactory area of performance, try to handle the subject in positive terms. Dwell on the kind of performance you would *like* to see, the goals you would like to reach.

7. Let the individual analyze and discuss her own deficiencies and let her

formulate her own plans for improvement. Those plans should be formulated during the interview and not left until later, if possible. With a little prompting from you, the employee will probably come to the same conclusions you came to before the interview.

8. In working out plans for future improvement, set very specific goals with specific time targets. The exact kinds of behavior to be expected in the future should be defined, and a definite time stated by which the new standards should be attained. In setting these time goals, keep in mind that nobody attains perfection. Make it clear to your employee that you don't expect perfection.

9. Allow the employee to air his or her own grievances fully.

10. Don't discuss salary in specific terms at the same time as the performance appraisal. To do this would distract attention from the subjects you want to focus on. Imply that salary review will provide an opportunity later to reward satisfactory achievement of the objectives set at the performance appraisal interview.

THE FOURTH "P" OF PRACTICE MANAGEMENT: OFFICE PROCEDURES

Most imperative for management in office procedures is "controlled accuracy." Nothing is more harmful in your practice life than errors. They generate ill will and possible legal actions. Errors arise out of lack of controls and non-coordination among responsible parties. Errors most noticeable to your patients usually will involve money rather than health.

We recommend that you follow a basic rule adhered to by accountants: *Delegate the various financial functions to more than one person so that a system of checks and balances becomes established naturally.* Such a system will also be a deterrent to embezzlement. The physician who reviews financial transactions daily won't be the one "ripped off."

Office procedures are accomplished best when systems are simple. ("K I S S"—"Keep it simple, sir.") Simple controls allow for less chance of error.

Consider that modern office machines can make jobs easier to learn and quicker to perform, and eliminate human errors. Heed this maxim: "If a machine can do a task, the machine should be doing it." Human labor is far more expensive and makes more mistakes than automated labor. Besides, the use of machines more often than not lets you keep a more perceptive eye on practice income and disbursements.

How to Keep Your Eye on Practice Income

Payment for services rendered should have individual patient entries made in a separate daily log—not the appointment book. Stay on the *cash* basis of accounting. For tax purposes record actual income rather than services dispensed. In contrast, reporting services rendered, even those not yet paid, would be the *accrual* basis of accounting.

To keep your eye on practice production enter the services rendered broken down into the type of service irrespective of whether it was paid for or not. This log entry will be your primary source of documentation for further entry onto individual accounting and billing cards. This allows for later management review. Record income in the daily log including mail receipts and direct patient payments. Issue prenumbered carbon copied receipts to patients and indicate "check" or "cash" as the manner of payment.

Deposit all income daily into the bank with no cash withdrawal, petty cash, or change funding allowed. Enter the total of the day's income in your monthly ledger. You should review and initial each day sheet and compare it with the appointment book. The bank deposit slip must agree with the day sheet income. These various ways of keeping your eye on practice income will be tools by which you can untangle financial matters in your office when the accountant or management consultant comes in to look over your books.

Unfortunately, it is in this daily check-up accounting area that many physicians abandon their personal responsibilities in managing the practice. They tend to excuse themselves from direct attention to basic accounting and leave it to an employee to determine if the day sheets agree with the posting to the patient's account cards. The result must inevitably be poor general office procedures, repeated errors and sometimes embezzlement.

A physician who fails to know his production and income will have unhappy patients and employees. Still, there are easy accounting short cuts—systems that reduce the time and trouble connected with giving office procedures your full attention.

The peg board system has great advantages in keeping these various multiple records up to date. It cuts down on time spent posting. It reduces errors. Since it requires writing through carbon to make entries on various documents which include the day sheet, the patient's account card, a statement and a receipt for payment, not too much checking is needed. The peg board system offers a receipt that is vital because it acknowledges payment and is an excellent antiembezzlement control. Patients want receipts as documented evidence for their tax deductions.

How to Use the Multipart Service-Receipt (Peg Board)

Use of the multipart pegboard service-receipt in the professional office is a well-established technique of reducing paperwork. Control-o-fax, Box 778, Waterloo, Iowa 50704 supplied the information offered here, and if you wish more explanation, contact that office.

There are three common applications of the pegboard multipart service-receipt.

1. It provides copies to the patient for his personal record; to serve as the "Attending Physician's Statement" in the event a third party was contracted to reimburse the patient for all or part of the medical bill.
2. It can act as the insurance claim form.
3. It may accumulate "Attending Physician's Statement" information during

the patient's visit and thus facilitate completion of third-party claim forms.

There are three copies for the multipart service-receipt: White is the office file copy; yellow is the insurance copy; pink is the patient's personal copy.

In the sequence of posting, the following steps are carried out:

1. Align the multipart service-receipt on the first open posting line of the day sheet when the patient enters the office.
2. Post account name, previous balance, transaction number and the date.
3. Attach the service-receipt to the patient's medical record and route to the examination room.
4. The doctor indicates services rendered and notes diagnosis on the service-receipt, which is returned to the business office by the patient.
5. The posting line of the service-receipt is aligned over the patient's name on the day sheet, pressing the peg holes of the service-receipt over the alignment pegs of the posting board.
6. Turn back the top copy and align the account card under the pink copy. Cover the first open posting line of the ledger with the posting line of the service-receipt. Complete the posting line using the special posting pen.
7. Remove the service-receipt from the pegboard and distribute the copies as needed by the office and patient.

How to Keep Check on Cash Disbursements

Maintaining a record of cash disbursements is equivalent to keeping the second half of your account books.

Use a single entry bookkeeping system where there is no need for various categories of expenditures, debits and credits in different ledgers.

Make a chronological entry of checks written to acknowledge the date of payment, the payee, the check number, the amount paid and an extension of the amount paid under the column provided.

Total each column at the end of the month and find that the total of the first column equals the total of all the other columns in the extensions. You will then have a recording of the disbursements by category.

Your bookkeeper, business manager, or receptionist may be delegated to make check payments for invoices received during the month.

He or she should clip the check to the invoice for your perusal before check signing. If supplies are invoiced, you might review the specific inventory. Then sign the check. Write the number and date of payment on the invoice and file all these invoices in a classification that will make an invoice easy to find later.

As mentioned in Chapter One, file by the month rather than by supplier or alphabetically. The audit by an IRS agent is better countered with monthly aggregations of various invoices.

A pegboard system is a good counter measure to the IRS audit also. As you write the check on the pegboard, the carbonization onto the check register permits a one-time writing of the payee, the date and the amount paid. The rest of the recordings follow the same procedure as above.

Make use of a three-on-a-page checkbook which allows for a memo stub. You can then make note of the payment, the purpose of payment, the date, the payee and the running balance. This system of checkwriting can be accompanied by a payroll stub for check payments to a large number of employees.

Establish Accounts Receivable Control

Accounts receivable control begins on the first of the month when you add charges made during the subsequent month's period. Then subtract payments and/or adjustments so that the resulting balance agrees with the new tally of the accounts receivable at the end of the month.

Take into account any credit write-offs or bad debts. They will clearly stand out.

As a control, the outside agent who does the accounting will want to spot-check by reviewing every entry of a total day's financial activity for a different day each month picked at random.

A Petty Cash System for the Office

To initiate a petty cash accommodation for your office there is a simple way to do it and keep control. Draft a check from the practice in whatever amount would be convenient; perhaps $50. Cash the check and retain the money in a petty cash box. As money is needed for expenditures, write a voucher for each one. Subsequently, reimburse the petty cash by the amount of the total of the vouchers up to the amount you began with—$50.

For a change fund mechanism—to make change for patients' larger currency denominations—supply another predetermined amount that would be used for making change for various patient transactions or deliveries. Perhaps $20 in dollar bills and six $5 bills would be proper. That amount remains at the receptionist's desk at all times for purposes of making change.

REFERENCE FOR CHAPTER SEVEN

1. Lakein, Alan *How to Get Control of Your Time and Your Life*. New York: Peter H. Wyden, Inc., 1973.

chapter eight

Galvanizing Employees To Accelerate Income

A good manager is a man who isn't worried about his own career but rather the careers of those who work for him. My advice: Don't worry about yourself. Take care of those who work for you and you'll float to greatness on their achievements.

— H.S.M. Burns, president, Shell Oil Co., in *Men at the Top*, 1959.

Trusted employees will build you greater office income than any single action you can take yourself during the course of any single day.

Although you may start out with only one part-time or full-time medical office assistant, as your practice grows you will probably augment your office staff to include a registered nurse, a laboratory or X-ray technician, a receptionist, a bookkeeper and others with various skills, depending upon the type of work you do and your office needs.

We recommend that you delegate tasks connected with running your office to aides whom you have taken the time and trouble to train. Subsequently, do not tolerate employees who cannot keep up with their training. Grant authority to take action but make known that you hold aides accountable for their actions.

Donald L. Ankerholz, a management consultant practicing in Denver, Colorado, believes that physicians get into more difficulty by delegating too little to their assistants rather than too much. Ankerholz says that there are three major benefits for the physician in delegating responsibilities to staff people, especially to nursing assistants:

1. You free yourself of routine aspects of patient care in order to work on more serious cases.
2. You can see more patients and boost productivity.
3. You are able to practice medicine with more ease.

Dean Van Horn, management consultant of Minneapolis, Minnesota, suggests that physicians are often guilty of refusing to surrender complete control of irrelevant activities in their offices. Nondelegators among physicians do pay the price. They are beset with a high pile of insurance claim forms and reports to be written as a result, and practices of these nondelegating doctors do not grow.

Robert K. Murray of Professional Consulting Services, Inc. in Columbia, Missouri also mentions that do-it-yourself doctors find little time to devote to reading clinical journals or to attending necessary medical meetings.

Over and over again, management consultants like Murray, Van Horn, and Ankerholz see an impressive increase of income for their clients because of improved production when physicians yield and delegate duties. They give over responsibilities to their personnel and reap rewards.

Make no mistake, it is you who assumes the final responsibility for any activity that takes place in your office, but at least someone else relieves you of the task of carrying out the activity.

DELEGATING BY THE CLINICAL TASK CHECKLIST

With a nurse or technician taking charge of delegated tasks in the clinical handling of treatment or diagnosis, should there be a reduced fee to the patients? No, fee reduction is unnecessary.

Your presence on the premises, assuming the responsibility that the delegated clinical task is done correctly, is equivalent to your delivering the service.

We presume that you have trained your assistant to do the task the way you wish. He or she is your surrogate who works under your supervision. In the final analysis, almost any task can be delegated if it does not violate the medical practice act of the state in which you practice medicine. Medical society counsels are usually well-informed about this and can supply that information if you seek it.

A number of clinical tasks offer themselves for delegation. Which of the following are you willing to give over to your aides?

Physical Examination Tasks
- Obtain height and weight
- Take temperature
- Take blood pressure on initial visit
- Take blood pressure of hypertensive patients
- Give vision screening
- Give hearing screening
- Perform tonometry
- Take PAP smear only
- Perform pelvic exam and take PAP smear
- Perform proctoscopic examination
- Perform breast examination

Therapy Tasks
- Administer immunizations
- Administer IM medications

- Administer IV medications
- Perform ear irrigations
- Do physiotherapy
- Remove sutures
- Give patient instructions and education
- Do well-baby care
- Do bladder irrigations and dilations
- Do urethral dilations
- Do ankle taping
- Do dressing application
- Do cast removal
- Do allergy testing
- Do all prenatal care
- Do throat cultures
- Perform advanced first aid

History and Patient Contact Tasks
- Take and record routine elements of the history
- Take and record history of present illness
- Take and record elements of systemic review
- Provide telephone advice on routine medical questions
- Provide telephone advice on minor medical questions
- Schedule patients for office visit if aide thinks necessary
- Visit hospital for routine patient checks
- Visit nursing home for routine patient checks
- Visit patient's home to determine necessity of MD visit
- Order refill of prescriptions with doctor's permission
- Schedule appointments on referral cases without conferring with physician
- Make entries on medical records
- Retrieve information from medical records

Laboratory, X-Ray and Related Tasks
- Obtain and mount EKG tracings
- Obtain venous blood samples
- Procure urine sample
- Perform urinalysis
- Prepare urine for microanalysis
- Determine hemoglobin

- Determine hematocrit
- Perform blood counts and smears
- Perform pulmonary function test
- Perform Master 2-step test
- Perform cytology
- Perform pregnancy test
- Take routine X-rays
- Take all X-rays
- Develop X-rays

A CHECKLIST OF OFFICE TASKS WHICH CAN BE DELEGATED

- Answer the telephone
- Schedule patient appointments
- Maintain listing of telephone call backs
- Determine the nature of patient incoming calls
- Check for messages with answering service
- Dial outgoing calls for doctor
- Telephone pharmacists
- Return nonemergency patient calls for doctor
- Receive patients
- Register patient's arrival
- Communicate with "no show" patients
- Schedule appointments with detail men
- Schedule appointment with accountant
- Prepare thank you notes to referring patients
- Maintain doctor's personal appointment log
- Verify new patient credit information
- Prepare a daily work schedule (patient appointments)
- Conduct daily work schedule staff meeting
- Attend daily work schedule staff meeting
- Maintain laundry supply records
- Maintain equipment maintenance schedule
- Maintain patient annual physical reminder file
- Maintain periodic task reminder file
- Open the office
- Make coffee, tea, herb tea or other beverages

- Open, sort and distribute mail
- Order needed janitor services
- Do office housekeeping chores
- Quiet noisy children
- Renew magazine subscriptions
- Check doctor's bag and refill
- Make inventory and originate order for medical supplies
- Review and authorize medical supplies purchase order
- Make inventory and originate order for office supplies
- Review and authorize office supplies purchase order
- Make inventory and originate drug orders
- Review and authorize drug purchase orders
- Make arrangements for hospital admissions
- Pull medical records for all of today's appointments
- Talk to pharmaceutical representatives
- Prepare Blue Shield claim (patient information)
- Complete Blue Shield Claim (diagnosis and description of services)
- Review and sign Blue Shield claims
- Prepare Medicare claim (Patient information)
- Complete Medicare claim (diagnosis and description of services)
- Review and sign Medicare claim
- Prepare Workmen's Compensation form (patient information)
- Complete Workmen's Compensation form (diagnosis and description of services)
- Review and sign Workmen's Compensation form
- Prepare attending physician's statement (patient information)
- Complete attending physician's statement (diagnosis and description of services)
- Review and sign attending physician's statement
- File claim forms in suspense file until payment is received
- Follow up control procedure on old claims
- Telephone insurance company about unpaid claims
- Prepare letter to insurance company about unpaid claims
- Post payments from insurance company to patient ledger
- Dispose of any difference between patient bill and insurance company disbursements
- Endorse checks received from patients

- Handle disposition of patient "rubber checks"
- Prepare checks for overpayments to the order of the patient
- Determine what correcting entries are needed in patient ledgers
- Prepare patient ledger adjustment forms
- Maintain a petty cash fund
- Balance and replenish petty cash fund
- Check invoices from suppliers for discounts
- Prepare checks for doctor's signature
- Review and sign expense checks
- Record cash disbursements in daily journal
- Record all cash received in daily journal
- Prepare bank deposit slip
- Make bank deposit and obtain receipt
- Reconcile the bank balance
- Run a trial balance of accounts
- Prepare payroll checks
- Sign payroll checks
- Record payroll disbursements in ledger
- Deposit withholding tax and F.I.C.A. with bank
- Maintain a listing of office problems
- Schedule and assign unusual tasks
- Take corrective action on employee problems
- Conduct a salary review
- Compose correspondence (business and personal)
- Compose patient medical correspondence
- Edit draft of outgoing correspondence
- Type and prepare correspondence for mailing
- Determine fee reductions or adjustments
- Communicate fee adjustment to patient
- Conduct office staff training in new procedures

HAVING AN INVENTORY SYSTEM THAT ALLOWS NO WASTE

It falls to the assistant whom you designate as your "supply sergeant" to maintain an inventory system that allows no waste in purchasing. Before wasteless maintenance may come about, however, you have to install the suitable inventory controls.

It is not difficult to follow an easy, workable inventory system that allows no waste. Our contention is that you ought to buy no more of any item than you normally use in one year.

A medical office frequently has storage limitations, and medical techniques are constantly in change with new procedures. Therefore, you have to weigh the possible advantages of buying at a "bargain" price against the disadvantages of obsolescence.

Your local medical supply dealer may permit *contract buying;* i.e., buying at a predetermined price and shipping as you need so that your storage problem will no longer be troublesome. Ask the dealer for that arrangement.

Most materials that are subject to destabilization are dated in code by the manufacturer. Any reputable supplier will explain the manufacturer's code to prevent your purchasing and receiving material which could be short-dated.

A properly operating inventory system will aid your staff in purchasing more effectively. This avoids overhead waste due to supplies that are aged, overlooked, misplaced or duplicated.

The assistant responsible for ordering supplies should become familiar with their costs and bring to your attention any valuable deals being offered by suppliers. He or she will then be ordering supplies by brand names or by specifications, as a matter of course, to avoid improper shipments and unnecessary delays. Your office pocketbook will reap the benefit of inventory control.

Inventory control will also keep you aware of rising costs and make you conscious of the quantity of supplies that you use in any given period. There won't be a sudden and embarrassing shortage of something needed immediately either.

With time, the whole ordering system can become semiautomated. Then, you can concentrate on patient care, secure in the knowledge that your storage shelves have all the materials and supplies required for you to render such care satisfactorily.

How to Install Effective Inventory Control

Industry has set an example of effective inventory control quite applicable to a medical office. You can install a similar system. What follows is a description of what to do.

Remove all your existing supplies from cabinets and closets and prepare a 5" × 7" inventory card for each item. List the item classification, manufacturer and description, and keep these cards in an inventory control card file by product category. You might, for example, arrange the cards by groups of materials as paper goods, cements, tapes, bandages, etc.

Determine a minimum/maximum quantity level for each item. Attach a tag to the minimum quantity with a rubber band, and when the tag is broken, it will be time to reorder that material.

For instance, if you determine that you use six boxes of plaster of Paris splints a month, and you decide that for economy you will purchase two dozen boxes at a time, you would establish your maximum at twenty-four and your minimum at six. (Note: the minimum level should always allow for at least a two-week supply.) A tag is placed around the six boxes with a rubber band. It is important always to use the items that are not tagged first. As soon as you are left with only tagged goods, reorder immediately.

When you do order an item, enter the date ordered and the quantity ordered on the 5"×7" inventory control card and on the back of the tag. Keep these various minimum quantity tags in a small box until you receive the goods from your dealer. When the new goods come in, retag the minimum and place the merchandise in your supply room.

You might use color coding also, for indicating when you are nearing a shortage in supply. For example, if you reach the minimum quantity of a product, attach a *red* signal to the inventory control card for this item. *Crimpgraf*® plastic inserts make excellent color coding identification signals. The plastic insert will flag your need for an immediate reorder.

You could assign meanings to other Crimpgraf® colors:

Green – after your assistant places the order, leave the red signal on the inventory card and insert the green signal adjacent to it to avoid double ordering.

Orange – this could indicate that you have received a back order slip from the supplier and orange would replace the red and green signals.

Blue – this could show that you have returned the product for credit. The blue signal will remain in place until you receive the credit invoice.

A Case Study of Inventory Control

Let us follow your "supply sergeant" as he or she monitors a shipment of three boxes of tongue depressors from the time the shipment arrives at your office to when it must be reordered:

1. The assistant checks the shipment against the invoice to insure that the proper number of pieces of the correct item have been received.

2. The assistant checks the price of tongue depressors on the invoice against the price recorded previously on the inventory file card to ascertain that no errors have been made. Any price change should be brought to your attention so that you can exercise your option to return the material. The assistant should change the item cost on the inventory card, only after verifying the price change from the dealer.

3. With an adding machine or calculator, the assistant confirms that the items listed in the invoice are correctly totalled. This step has been eliminated on computerized invoices used by most suppliers.

4. The assistant then attaches an inventory control tag to the minimum quantity of tongue depressors—in this case one box. The date and quantity received are entered on the 5"×7" file card. If there is any back order number it is entered on the same file card.

5. The assistant then stores the boxes of tongue depressors in the supply closet, placing the tagged box in the rear.

DO YOU HAVE ALL THE EQUIPMENT YOU NEED?

You can have nonproductive office time—a waste—by lacking essential equipment.

Case in Point: Orthopedic surgeon Alex Kimbrow of Madison, Wisconsin, wasted much time by not having an office X-ray machine. If a patient came to him with a swollen foot, for instance, Kimbrow couldn't diagnose the problem immediately without the benefit of a radiograph. He would have to send the patient to a hospital for a diagnostic film. The hospital went through a time-consuming procedure and supplied the radiologist's report in thirty-six hours. The patient had to return for another appointment for proper treatment. If a cast was required, the patient would have undergone a great deal of discomfort in the interim.

Kimbrow finally recognized his need and acquired an X-ray unit, which made money for him and saved him time.

AVOIDING NONPRODUCTIVE OFFICE TIME

Thomas A. Edison once said, "Waste is worse than loss. The time is coming when every person who lays claim to ability will keep the question of waste before him constantly."

The key to your profitable practice is how you manage office time to milk the most production from each minute.

Published charts show that the average physician spends only 50 percent of his time in direct "hands on" patient care. The other 50 percent is spent in administrative work, driving to the hospitals, reading medical charts, making and receiving telephone calls, personal business and other similar items. The important thing is that typically, a large portion of your attention is given over to other actions besides patient care when patient care is the only thing you sell.

You may do an excellent job of managing efficient "hands on medicine" by working at a fast pace. This is not generally the area in which you need production improvement. Thus, seeing more patients per day is not so much a matter of spending less time with each patient as it is spending less time *between* patients with nonpatient care activities.

It is somewhat difficult in fact, to waste time and motion in the one-to-one doctor-patient relationship even though some physicians normally work at a faster pace than do others.

Waste prevention should come instead in situations where patients are not directly involved such as the too long coffee break at the hospital in the morning, the interesting but unproductive chatting with nurses and the medical assistants, the unnecessary travel and a late start in the morning. No one expects you to be inhuman and drive yourself relentlessly, but by carefully reviewing your daily activities you could quickly pinpoint a number of waste-preventing actions to take.

Because medicine is a very personal service and your productivity is largely measured by the procedures that you perform, management of your time is certainly a major key to profitable practice.

Eleven Waste-Preventing Actions

Consequently, we recommend that you set into motion the following eleven waste-preventing actions and add more of them of your own invention.

1. Have your employee telephone "no show" patients ten minutes after their appointment times to see what has happened to them. If a "no show" misses two appointments without furnishing an acceptable reason, you should no longer accept him as your patient.

2. Similarly, patients who always arrive late for appointments should be told that the appointment time is to be taken seriously. After four infractions of your scheduling, weed out the chronic late arriver.

3. Arrange office hours to meet community needs such as holding evening hours two days a week.

4. Allow ample time for various types of visits such as first visits, checkups, physical examinations and particular procedures.

5. Do not make conflicting appointments or overcrowd the schedule.

6. Allow two or three short periods for catching your breath or resting throughout the day.

7. When it is necessary to refuse a patient an appointment, always explain why.

8. When an emergency takes you out of the office, have your assistant explain the situation to waiting patients and give them the choice of waiting or returning at another time.

9. If you must cancel appointments, explain why and notify the patient in advance, if possible, to make a new appointment.

10. Use an intercommunication system within your office to save employees and yourself from walking from room to room when seeking assistance.

11. Use automated equipment everywhere you can such as the dictating machine, the electric thermometer, the electric adding machine or a calculator, a photocopy machine, an electric typewriter, microfilming records, the purchase of your own telephone equipment, a checkwriter and a postage meter, especially the postage meter type that seals the envelope at the same time that it stamps it.

chapter nine

What Every Profit-Minded Doctor Should Know About Setting Fees And Collecting Bills

Money is like a sixth sense — and you can't make use of the other five without it.

— Somerset Maugham, *The New York Times*, October 18, 1958

E. A. "Bud" Thieman, a professional business consultant, head of the Service Bureau for Doctors in Louisville, Kentucky, noticed an astonishing occurrence about fee complaints received years ago, before the present rate of inflation.

Thieman had a surgeon client who shared space with a younger physician. The young man often assisted him at surgery. The surgeon paid this young doctor $15 for his assistance, and tacked a $15 charge onto the patient's bill. So, if the normal fee for a procedure was $100, the surgeon would charge $115; if the fee usually was $200, the surgeon would charge $215.

The surgeon heard hardly any grumblings from patients concerning the $115 and $215 bills but got plenty of complaints from his $100 and $200 bills. The circumstances were so striking that Thieman make a detailed study of the grumblings. His findings: the surgeon had received twelve times as many complaints about the $100 fees as about the $115.

These results caused Thieman to persuade a number of other physicians to quote fees in odd amounts. After a few years of experience, he could name the figures that produced the most patient resistance, and those that produced the least.

For smaller cases, he found that figures ending with $1, $2, $3, $4, $6, $7, $8 and $9 were more acceptable than $5, $10, $15, and other rounded-off numbers that went all the way up to $98. Numbers like $104, $106, and $108 met with less resistance than $100 for the same service.

Going higher, Thieman found the preferable figures to be $110, $115, $135, $165, $185, $195, $210, $215, $235, $265, $285, $295, and so on, up to $500. The undesirable figures were $50, $75, $100, $125, $175, $200, $250, $275, $300, etc.

Really high figures could be rounded off to the hundred dollars—as long as it was an "odd" hundred dollars. In other words, a physician could charge $600,

$700, $800, $900, $1,200, $1,600 and $1,800 without hearing grumblings. But numbers $1,000, $1,500, and $2,000 were much less acceptable to patients. The pattern continued all the way up; a $3,300 fee was more readily accepted than a $3,000 fee for the same service.[1]

Thieman's experience is a classic story told by practice management consultants. It probably would take the collective wisdom of a dozen psychologists to find the reasons for this true finding. The results are conclusive, however; odd fees are best for you and your patient.

CHARGING THE FAIREST WAY

We recommend that you charge by the minute rather than by the routine. If a standard fee in your office, for instance, is $16 for a ten-minute office visit, and your patient requires twenty minutes of your attention, your fee should be $32. The office visit in that instance was obviously not a standard one, and your charge should not be standard.

Important: William H. Kidd, a former president of the Society of Medical-Dental Management Consultants, who practices in Raytown, Missouri, backs us up. He suggests that the usual physician is not time-conscious enough. One of Kidd's jobs as a management consultant is to make his client aware of how much time he is actually spending with each patient, then charge accordingly. Otherwise, when the doctor goes ahead and makes an across-the-board increase in fees, he is being unfair to the patient who requires less time.

When you use the management consultant's services to evaluate your overhead, you will finally arrive at a "turnkey" hourly cost. His evaluation will take into account your fixed and variable costs and your average expenses comparable to others in your specialty. Then the consultant quantifies earnings against expenses and computes your fee rate per minute.

Important: James A. Tipping, management consultant from Wheaton, Illinois, suggests that you remind yourself of your primary responsibility—patient care—and if the patient needs your attention or insists on taking your time, you are justified in making an extra charge for that care. Conversely, if you digress and wish to spend extra time visiting without medical justification, you won't be justified in making an extra charge.

Tipping offers a word of caution: repeated interruptions by telephone calls or nurse's questions about other patients during the patient's private time with you will justify that patient's feeling your attention has been diluted. Then, setting your fee purely on a time basis will be grossly unfair. You will be charging your patient inordinately, and he will know it.

Using the Charge Ticket

The best way to establish and inform your patient of office fees is with the *charge ticket*.

The charge ticket is a slip that you hand your patient for delivery to the receptionist. The patient's charge ticket may designate the various services you have rendered, the charge for each service, and the total fee for all of them that visit.

Albert T. Wakelee, a management consultant from Buffalo Grove, Illinois, has expressed concern that most physicians do not charge for all the services they render. For instance, an injection may not be billed because you failed to mark on the ticket that you gave one.

He suggests that a pelvic examination is a good example of "telescoping" fees; i.e., lumping fees for a number of services together under one heading. The telescoping of services under one quoted fee is not an acceptable practice anymore in our present consumer-conscious society.

DO YOUR SERVICES COST TOO MUCH?

According to a nationwide survey by pollster Louis Harris, medical consumers have changed their opinion about physicians.

Medicine was our country's most respected profession in 1966, but it has taken a nosedive since then. From 72 percent of Americans then voicing the opinion that they have a "great deal of confidence" in their doctors, today less than 45 percent express the same degree of trust.

One of the public's major peeves is expressed by the patient's monetary bleat: "You cost too much! While I was in the hospital you popped in, glanced at my chart, asked me a question or two, and popped out. The whole visit took ninety seconds and you charged for a full visit! You cost too much!"

The patient's cry may have its origin in an attitude brought about by physicians who do not discuss their fees. By failing to mention them at all, doctors convey their feelings of guilt about the size of their fees. They are shrugging off any responsibility to explain billings and what they include and that these are usual and customary charges in the medical community.

You should be ready at all times to explain the reasons for the charges you make. Just as you treat the patient's ills, you have to be ready to treat the patient's monetary complaints. The result will be happier thereby, than if you offer no explanation at all.

Case in Point: Dr. Scott C. Rieger of South Holland, Illinois, relatively new in practice at the time, submitted a bill to his patient who plainly showed her attitude that she considered the fee excessive. Recognizing his responsibility to explain the bill, Rieger contacted the patient and was very specific as to the reasons why his fee was what had been submitted. About a week later the disgruntled patient turned around and referred another patient to the doctor. His explanation had been well-received. Today, more than three years since the initial confrontation, the patient continues to refer other patients and is obviously a well-satisfied patient.

We believe that it is naive for you to think it unprofessional to discuss money matters with your patient. Fees hold equal importance for both of you. All of us know of doctors who build their own problems by reciting with a wink of the eye, "Oh, don't worry about it. It will be OK!" These doctors do themselves a disservice and cause their own overabundance of accounts receivable (a/c) by their attitude of shirking fee discussions.

HOW TO PRESENT YOUR FEE

Because some physicians have found fee presentation inhibiting and an obstacle in their relationship with patients, they put off the task of telling how much a procedure will cost and how it can be paid. The result is predictable—invariably the patient is shocked when he sees the bill. The physician loses hero status in his patient's eyes even if life or limb had been saved by the doctor.

Presentation of your fee is one of those inevitables best met by stating it openly. Everyone knows that you run a medical practice with one of its purposes being to earn you a living. Therefore, reveal your fee. In most instances, whatever is the extent of their financial circumstances, patients want to know their obligations in order to reduce them where they can.

> *Case in Point:* A patient called family practice specialist Irving Meyerson of Grand Rapids, Michigan, at 3 o'clock on a frozen, rainy morning. The emergency telephone call awakened the doctor from a deep sleep and caused him to struggle out of bed, pull on his clothes, huddle into the cold car and finally get it started.
>
> The patient lived miles across town, and it took the haggard physician nearly an hour to get there, sliding sideways over the ice most of the way. When at last he arrived and examined the girl who was ill, he discovered she had nothing more than a severe cold.
>
> "Why didn't you call me in the daytime?" Meyerson inquired.
>
> "We're not rich people, Doc, and not able to pay much," the father explained, "so we thought we'd call when you weren't too busy."

Three Steps to Stating Your Fees Without Feeling Guilt

To get over the bugaboo of feeling guilty when you state your fee, we suggest you approach the subject in three steps:

First, query your patient about doubts and questions that have him feeling anxious or depressed. Provide him with as much medical information about his condition and the treatment as you deem beneficial. Telling these medical facts will relax you, since you will have command of an area that you know well.

Second, ask the patient to repeat what he understands about the diagnosis and the prime prognostic hazard. Prompt him with more information to fill in the gaps in his knowledge. Get him to accept the treatment plan you have outlined and ask for his confirmation that he will follow that plan by cooperating faithfully.

Third, say words that follow this line of thought:

"Now, Mr. Patient, the only things that could possibly be concerning you are how long treatment will take, what it will cost, and how you plan to pay for it. Is that true?

SETTING FEES AND COLLECTING BILLS

"The treatment which you have agreed we must go through to get you feeling better will take six visits over four months and will entail some laboratory tests. Each visit will cost $60 except the first which costs $125. The total fee is $425.

"You have told me about your personal situation. I believe it will probably be most satisfactory for you to pay this bill by making an initial payment of $125 and four regular monthly payments of $75 each. Will that be satisfactory?"

Take Note: This little speech involves a breakdown of the fee into units. The patient is fully informed of what he is paying for in its telling.

There is no pause after you have stated the total fee in order to carry the patient immediately to a discussion of the payment arrangement. He will not question the extent of the fee for services which "you have agreed we must go through to get you feeling better . . ." His problem is, "How shall I pay the fee?"

THE ONGOING BATTLE OVER FEES

Battles over fees will usually occur because of your patient's determination that his illness was not cured or his surgery had a bad result. Then he will blame you and balk at paying for something that he finds unsatisfactory. Nonpayment is the main form of punishing the doctor that a patient has at his command.

If you could look inside your patient's mind it might surprise you to discover what he thinks about your service, your office, your charges, your staff, and other things. It is easy to misjudge patients by incorrectly estimating what they could pay or by believing they hold medicine in higher regard than they do.

Publilius Syrus said: "A small debt produces a debtor; a large one, an enemy."

Getting occasional deadbeat patients to pay on their overdue accounts is an unhappy circumstance of the ongoing battle over fees. There are very few offices that have no patients who are delinquent in making payments. Although 90 percent of patients do not need prompting with paying bills, some need a lot of prompting.

It becomes clear that a main responsibility of your staff is to identify the 2 or 3 percent of the patient population in your office who are outright deadbeats. Your office manager or bookkeeper will usually be the responsible employee to make that identification and follow up with stiff collection procedures.

Surprisingly, a follow-up on the delinquency sometimes will actually bring the patient back into your office for subsequent examination. He or she may have experienced new signs and symptoms which were not present at the initial visit. Repeated personal phone calls and letters are needed to accomplish this return or payment.

The delinquent patient is very much like an unruly child who wants to be disciplined by the doctor authority. Unfortunately, Marcus Welby, M.D. is the only physician we know who treated only one patient per week and therefore had the luxury of much follow-up time. Your business manager will have to fill in for you as the authority figure.

The battle goes on! Collections must be attempted and made. Your collector has to be a counselor, investigator, salesperson, public relations representative, father confessor, and a student of human nature all rolled into one. Collecting is a challenging facet of managing a medical practice. It is governed by certain essentials of credit economics through which most Americans acquire what they want when they want it and pay for it out of future earnings.

In the case of medical care, the word *need* may be substituted for the word *want*. Unlike the obtaining of consumer goods, the acquisition of medical services more often will be budgeted not according to income and the convenience of payments, but by the patient's physical, mental and emotional needs.

CHANGING TIMES FOR HEALTH CARE CREDIT

In today's consumer market, the attitude toward credit is becoming more formalized simply because during the past decade there has been an abuse by consumers of planned purchasing by orderly and moral procedures. The familiar monthly charge account has been the accepted modern way of buying household and personal goods and services. Various kinds of installment payment plans have provided convenient methods of buying homes, cars, home furnishings, appliances and other things. Families could pay little or no interest for the privilege of deferred payment. This was often the only possible method of buying.

Times have changed! We live in a society of credit cards—the "plastic world." Payment of the monthly charge account is expected when the bill is received and if it is not made, a finance charge of 1 percent or 1½ percent interest per month is tacked on.

More and more people are coming to expect finance charges to be added onto their health care bills, too. The professional person is also beginning to look upon finance charges as an additional source of income. A physician should not be in the credit business, but often he is. Medical services and patient care should be his only sources of income, but unfortunately they are not.

The physician who has painted himself into a corner by allowing too liberal a policy of deferred payments by his patients has been forced to seek advice from financial institutions specializing in collections. In the following subsections, we have summarized some of the recommendations made by banks, finance companies, credit managers and various credit and collection experts for medical services. How to create an efficient collection system and thrive on fee-for-service in your practice is our theme.

YOUR OFFICE POLICY IN BUSINESS MATTERS

Your first requirement in having a creative collection system is to establish and enforce an office policy in business matters. What this means is that you decide beforehand, in discussions with your business manager and other office assistants who might be involved in credit or collection, what must be done in these credit and collection matters.

The policy should include who is to enforce the rules and how they are to be carried out. Set flexible rules but establish definite guidelines. Judgment will be the order of the day and when in doubt, personnel should discuss various collection problems with you.

Accordingly, record the office policy in your office manual, which we have described in Chapter One. Leave nothing to chance and allow no guesswork. The recorded policy ought to explain your overall philosophy governing the business side of medical practice on your premises. It will set forth a step-by-step procedure in doing the collection work.

Collecting needs to be accomplished in order that all staff members and the doctor can take home earnings to live on. The collection policy in your office will be a payment plan for dispensers of medical services as well as the recipients. No collections, no take-home pay! That is a rule you might consider enforcing.

THE FOUR "Cs" OF A PATIENT CREDIT APPLICATION

Modern collection techniques can shrink your accounts receivable to less than 2 percent of gross billings if your credit and collection procedures take into account the four "Cs" of credit analysis. These include "Capital," the patient's general financial resources; "Capacity," the patient's earning ability and steady employment; "Character," the patient's general reputation and moral standing; and "Conditions," the general economic, social and personal atmosphere at the time.

Much of this credit analysis will be accomplished simply from a look at a credit application which the individual is asked to fill out in your office. An application appraisal will help you or your business manager or the particular person in your office who handles financial matters to make a credit decision about the new patient.

Important: The patient's credit application is as important to your financial health as the patient's case history is to his physical health.

Use of the credit application in advance of rendering medical service is a way of getting your bills paid on an equal par with other creditors. It is not unusual for a person to pay his stack of monthly bills with the doctor's statement taken off the top and slipped to the bottom. You are likely to be the doctor who must wait until other creditors are satisfied simply because they levy monthly finance charges, and you may not. The fear of repossessions and extra interest added to other bills for tangible goods makes for chronic abuse of medical credit.

Regular income from the dispensing of service keeps you in practice. That is obvious. Not as well recognized is the fact that you can guarantee you will receive a greater percentage of the fees you earn by getting fuller credit information before you actually examine the patient. We heartily advise that you know the person prior to "laying on hands" for medical treatment.

What the Credit Application Should Reveal

A familiar slogan among consumer credit associations is "an account well opened is already half collected." This means simply that your office manager should obtain all the credit information essential for office records at the beginning of the physician-patient relationship. Certainly, some of the information will overlap with data taken for case records and, therefore, the patient or the patient's guardian can be asked to fill out a single detailed form.

To have an efficient collection system from the very beginning of your patient contact, the following information about the individual is generally considered necessary for adequate credit investigation and for collection purposes:

1. Name of patient, and the name of the guardian if the patient is not an adult.
2. Marital status of adult patient and name of spouse, if any.
3. Home and business addresses and telephone numbers of patient, or of parent or guardian.
4. Patient's or guardian's place of employment, the address and present position.
5. Name of nearest relative and relationship, other than husband or wife.
6. Health insurance applicable to present or future care.
7. Name and address of person or organization financially responsible for the account.
8. Name of person recommending patient.

As an office policy, some business managers include required information about the patient's charge accounts, since these are fine indices for a credit evaluation. We suggest that you *not* ask for bank account information and *do not* take superficial signs of wealth as a way of guessing at the individual's prosperity.

HOW TO USE YOUR COMMUNITY CREDIT BUREAU

We recommend that you obtain a credit bureau report on every patient to whom credit is to be extended. This may be done even before you meet the patient for the first time in a doctor-patient relationship. Certainly, when a substantial sum for your services is involved and there is some question as to the patient's credit, you should check his credit rating with the local credit bureau.

A community credit bureau usually provides a range of reporting services depending upon the depth of information you contract to purchase. The credit bureau's report will answer many questions asked by the four "Cs" of credit analysis, especially *capital* and *capacity* and another one: *paying habits*. Practically all persons who have used credit in your community will have a payment record and credit history stored in the credit bureau's files. It is the best avenue of information on new credit customers and new residents, for it can scan the entire country and gather information from other bureaus.

SETTING FEES AND COLLECTING BILLS 159

The cost of membership and fee per credit report is quite modest. For example, the Stamford Credit Rating Bureau, Inc. of Stamford, Connecticut (reporting May 14, 1980), charges $35 annually for a membership plus $1.23 state tax. When you telephone for an immediate credit rating while your new patient is seated in your reception room filling out various forms, etc., that verbal report costs $1.50.

An employee of the Credit Rating Bureau locates the appropriate file jacket, which holds full credit information about your prospective patient, and reads you everything in there. You can check with other local creditors (called "revising") to get a more personal payment history on the person. In the file also will be information about when the individual was entered, which other creditors in town have made checks, how much the person owes around town, when others last called for credit checks, and what is the patient's credit rating such as A-1, R-1, O-1, etc. which may decipher down to "good," "better," "best" or "poor," "poorer," "worst."

Incidentally, if no credit report is available for a person, since the bureau has no file jacket on him, that fact is important too. You will be creating a first entry for the individual.

The Stamford Credit Rating Bureau charges $1 for a report on "no file." If you check on out-of-town patients and go "foreign," the fee is an extra $1.50.

Stamford also has a collection department in its credit rating bureau that works on the basis of no collection, no fee. For a bill collected of under $25 the fee is one half; for a bill collected of over $25 the fee is one-third. For out-of-state "skips," the fee is one-half. If the account is sent to an attorney with your approval the fee is one-half. A creditor does not have to be a member of the Stamford Credit Rating Bureau, which can be considered a typical credit bureau operation, to make use of its collection department. We will discuss the use of collection agencies a little later in this chapter.

Recommendation: You should use a community credit rating bureau because the American public is seemingly always on the move, and no matter where a person relocates, his credit record is almost sure to follow him. Credit bureaus interchange credit information constantly. They have national and even international networks.

The credit bureau report read to you over the telephone allows your business manager to make an immediate judgment, in consultation with you, as to just how much time and attention you might choose to invest in that new patient.

Additionally, the credit bureau sends you a written report that can be attached to the new patient's medical registration. You will know without a shadow of a doubt if a new patient has the ability and the willingness to pay his obligations. That way, you will be able to avoid giving extensive treatment to deadbeats.

NINE DANGER SIGNALS OF DEADBEATS

The credit application that you ask the new patient to fill out will become your most valuable tool in spotting a deadbeat in advance. According to Rudolph

M. Severa, formerly Secretary-Treasurer of the Associated Credit Men of New York, there are nine advance danger signals that flag a deadbeat when you analyze his application for credit in your office. These are:

1. Residence in a rooming house or other domicile for transients.
2. Suspected minors, alchoholics, drug addicts and mental patients.
3. No prior history or too much prior history with excessive numbers of creditors.
4. Foreign nationals, divorced people who are not self-supporting, retirees with no evidence of income.
5. Racketeers, carnival workers, fortune tellers, and traveling salesmen with short lengths of service in out-of-town companies.
6. People (such as prostitutes) who live under undesirable circumstances or who cannot supply financial references.
7. People who rent only desk space or telephone service and have no bank reference.
8. Workers who live on fees earned at home, such as music teachers, tutors, and masseurs; or workers in shady businesses.
9. Any person for whom it is impossible to obtain a prior history.

Charles A. Crane, manager of a New Jersey collection agency, says, "There is no stereotyped deadbeat. The best heeled patient in your practice might turn out to be the toughest account to collect."

THE BEST COLLECTION PROCEDURE FOR SLOW-PAYING PATIENTS

As we have said, except for outright deadbeats, most patients will welcome any help you offer to rid them of their financial obligations.

Believe it or not, you are actually doing your patients a favor by encouraging pay-as-you-go treatment. Most people are prepared to pay for routine office visits but often leave the office without paying simply because no one gave them an opportunity to do so. Yes, odd as it may sound, patients do not pay for visits immediately because nobody asks for payment!

Your office policy should include having the receptionist say to the patient preparing to leave your office, "Are you going to take care of the charge today (and the unpaid balance as well)?"

She should say this while standing expectantly, at her desk, receipt book in hand. This is the time when the patient is reminded of the specific payment arrangements he has made with you or your business manager. He must take action—pay or make an excuse. Often, it is easier to pay.

If the patient is of the slow-paying type and offers only a partial amount that falls short of what was promised, your receptionist should follow up with the question, "Will you add today's balance for a greater payment on your next visit?"

SETTING FEES AND COLLECTING BILLS

The obvious answer must be "Yes." What if there are no more visits? That is when your office must start billing that excuse-giving slow payer.

How to Carry Out Cyclical Billing

Cyclical billing is the best method to use for sending out statements. This kind of regular billing is an essential part of a good collection procedure. Punctuality in billing encourages prompt payment by jogging the patient's memory about his financial obligation. Therefore, we feel an emphasis on regular cyclical billing is necessary; otherwise, you will not be receiving full compensation for all the professional services rendered.

Cyclical billing divides the patient account cards into equal groupings and spreads the billing for these groups throughout the month. For example, patients with last names beginning with A to G could be billed in the first week on an inactive Wednesday; H to N might be billed the second week, etc. This will reduce the peak load at month's end and allows for a more even flow of income during the month.

Cyclical billing makes it routine to follow up on delinquencies the next month when they become apparent at their slotted billing time and are not jammed together with all billing at month's end.

Divisions for billing cycles will be decided by how large your practice is and how many patients you have on the books. It may be determined by the type of billing system you employ as well.

There are two types of billing systems to choose from: the manual and the computerized.

The manual billing system is prepared either through a pegboard, with the patient's statement individually typed, carbon copied, photocopied or printed by bookkeeping machine.

The computerized billing system is accommodated by in-house control with a computer on the premises or through a centralized billing agency to whom you send your accounts.

The best type to choose from the various combinations for the majority of practices seems to be photocopied manual billing. It keeps the responsibility of collection where it belongs—in your office and out of the hands of unknowing outsiders who might offend patients.

You can do up to 10,000 billings a month with a cyclical manual photocopy system.

The Best Billing Procedure

A statement saying "For professional services" is no longer acceptable in this age when patients have health insurance companies and other third party carriers insisting upon itemized bills.

The best billing procedure is to itemize charges on the first statement. Have your billing clerk write statements with the dollar sign and zeros omitted. Show the month during which each service was performed and clearly mark follow-up statements as "second statement" or "third statement."

The collection timetable that your office uses may include:

First month – Send statement.

Second month – Send statement.

Third month – Send collection letter number one.

Fourth month – Send collection letter number two or make telephone call.

Third week of Fourth month – Send collection letter number three.

Fifth month – Send collection letter number four which notifies the patient that since he has ignored all communications, the account is being turned over to a collection agency.

SAMPLES OF EFFECTIVE COLLECTION LETTERS

Rather than sticking clever labels on statements and other commercial devices to attract attention to an overdue bill, a more personal approach is the best way to stimulate a slow-paying patient to settle his bill. We furnish here a series of six letters to keep your message in front of the slow payer. Each letter lets the debtor know that it is necessary to get his financial obligation out of the way.

COLLECTION LETTER NUMBER ONE

> You have not responded to our previous request for payment. Please remit at this time or contact us if there are any questions remaining regarding your account.

COLLECTION LETTER NUMBER TWO

> When we wrote you recently you apparently failed to understand that payment or a definite arrangement was expected. This account has been overdue several months. We ask that you remit now.

COLLECTION LETTER NUMBER THREE

> We have been expecting word from you about your now overdue account. We do not wish to embarrass you by giving your account to a collector, and it should not be necessary. Please get in touch with us at once so that arrangements can be made to suit your circumstances.

COLLECTION LETTER NUMBER FOUR

> You have been given opportunities to contact us about your long overdue account. We believe that every courtesy has been extended to you. Unless we hear from you within ten days we shall place this account in the hands of a collector for enforced action.

COLLECTION LETTER NUMBER FIVE FOR A PARTIAL PAYMENT

> We appreciate your partial payment; however, in view of the overdue nature of your account we respectfully ask that you contact this office so an understanding of your payment plan may be established.

COLLECTION LETTER NUMBER SIX FOR AN INSURANCE PAYMENT

> Your health insurance company has remitted (insert the amount) payment on your account. This leaves a balance of (insert the amount). As you know, the amount that the insurance company pays is between you and the insurance company. The doctor provided the service to you and you are responsible for the bill. May we expect a payment on the balance of your account now?

HOW TO FOLLOW UP DELINQUENT ACCOUNTS

In following delinquent accounts we strongly encourage that there be some indication on the patient account card as to what action was taken. Record when letters were sent and telephone calls were made, who was contacted, and what were the promises made.

We think you ought not to make you own collection calls. Telephone calls made by your business manager or someone other than you will be more effective. They give the patient a chance to save face by letting the caller hear him out. He will likely have a logical excuse for not paying the bill. Slow payers usually do.

There are four basic principles that your caller can apply in the use of the telephone for bill collection:

1. Speak clearly.
2. Control the voice volume.
3. Use the right voice tone and attitude.
4. Control the rate of speech.

Collections by telephone demand a combination of credit knowledge, communications skill, and an understanding of people. Does your collection caller fit that description?

The best way to institute telephone collections as a procedure of your office policy is to first set up a collection headquarters within the office. It should be a private place that contains a telephone, credit records, an organizing call plan, pencil, and paper.

The caller must know the principles of telephone communication and be skilled in the use of language.

Prompt and precise follow-up on any promise made by the patient to pay at a certain time is mandatory. Your collection caller must exhaust all possible means of contacting the delinquent party and complete each contact with a definite understanding and commitment by that person. When satisfactory arrangements have been made, note on the ledger card the arrangement made and notify the doctor. That should be part of the office policy.

EIGHT GUIDELINES IN SELECTING A COLLECTION AGENCY

A professional collection agency is quite useful after you have attempted but failed to collect an outstanding account for six months. However, guidelines are needed in selecting an agency which will not be offensive and tarnish your professional image.

Here are eight guidelines to aid you in selecting a collection agency:

1. Check your local medical society and heed its advice as to the reliability of that agency.
2. Check with the local Chamber of Commerce or Better Business Bureau and ask for a reference for that agency.
3. Run a credit check on the owner of the agency and on the agency itself. Find out if they are financially responsible and well-established.
4. Check with the Medical/Dental Hospital Bureaus of America, or the Associated Credit Bureau of America to learn if that agency is a member and if it conforms to the high standards of operation.
5. Find out the kind of collection methods used. Ask the agency manager to show you the reminders and follow-up pieces mailed. A reputable agency will welcome such a request.
6. Ask for the percentage of accounts collected and the agency's fees for the various ages of the accounts receivables submitted.
7. Ask for the names of other professional people who have used the agency's services and check with them to learn of their satisfaction.
8. As a general rule, do not sign a contract, since ethical agencies seldom use them.

SHOULD YOU TRY TO COLLECT BY LEGAL ACTION?

We counsel that you should not resort to the courts in trying to collect accounts receivable. It is a drastic step of limited value that is usually offset by resultant ill will and possible malpractice counterclaims against you.

Justified or not, a malpractice suit is a common retort by patients to physicians' attempts to collect. Many doctors delay even the thought of legal actions until after the statute of limitations expires. This statute in your state determines the extent of time during which a malpractice action can be filed. The interval varies from state to state.

We vote against any attempt to collect by legal action for several reasons. The patient who is vengeful will express his vengeance by holding back payment. He is just waiting for you to provoke him further. Why give him an additional motive to seek revenge for a real or imagined wrong done him?

The person who is unable to pay has no assets for your attorney to attach. Even if you win your case in court, it will be a study in frustration, since you will have won nothing financially. The old maxim says, "You can't get blood from a stone."

If you have a number of these accounts receivable that have brought you to this exasperated point where you are considering turning them over to a collection attorney, it is clear that your office is not doing its part in pursuing collections correctly. Something is wrong with your policy or the way you are executing it.

Any physician will usually have two months of accounts receivable on file. If many accounts are running three months and more past due, you should start reviewing your billing and collecting procedures. With modern collection techniques, you should be able to shrink your accounts receivable to 3 percent of your gross billings.

Collections requiring more drastic action, that run at a rate of 10 percent of billings in your office, are probably hampered by one or more of these problems:

- You are recording inadequate credit information.
- You are following incorrect collection procedures.
- You are pressing too hard for prompt payment and losing patients.
- You are failing to ask for payment firmly enough for fear of offending and losing the patient.

Make it part of your office policy that the total amount of your receivables will equal no more than the value of three months gross service which you ordinarily dispense. To check your collection ratio, it is simple to divide accounts receivable by one month of billing. If the quotient is greater than three, you are in trouble. The three-to-one ratio holds true for a general practitioner or the specialist in family practice. Other specialists such as surgeons, obstetricians, pediatricians, etc. should revise their ratios downward.

RECEIVING UP-FRONT FUNDING BY FACTORING

A standard business practice in many areas of retail trade and in dentistry is finding its way into medical practice management. In return for 10 percent of the money you receive for services performed, a factor will pay you cash for your accounts receivable.

In effect, you send your patient billings to a third party, the factoring house, and get up-front funding. This relieves you of collection headaches and provides a predictable cash flow each month. The billing function is handled by the factoring firm, discounted to pay its fee, and paid to you weekly without the many irregularities that frequently accompany monthly office collections.

> *Case in Point:* Suppose that the accounts open in your files at any particular moment are congealing. They amount to about $100,000. They range from dead and frozen accounts considered to be lost to newly billed ones of very satisfied patients. Lumped together, you will immediately receive approximately $50,000 for these accounts from the factoring company, less its 10 percent discount.
>
> The actual initial payout is determined by the overall age of your accounts receivable. The newer they are, the more money you will get for them. You receive the remaining money, less a percentage, as it is paid by patients to the factoring company. Thus, the difference between the amount you paid initially and the total value of all the receivables is withheld until patients pay their bills, a procedure known as "reserve accounts."
>
> Your patients, in the meantime, receive a letter from the factoring firm signed by you that says the firm is now handling billing and collection functions for your office. Individual patients have their payment procedures worked out with the factor. Perhaps a payment book is supplied to enforce the patient's promised schedule.[2]

In the event that you choose to use a factor, follow the same guidelines for selecting one that we suggested regarding using a collection agency.

REFERENCES FOR CHAPTER NINE

1. Thieman, E. A. "Your fee: odds or even?" *Dental Management,* June 1976.
2. Green, David. "Fast cash from factoring." *Dental Management,* December 1975.

chapter ten

Skyrocket Medical Practice Net Income by Budgeting Office Expense

Money itself isn't the primary factor in what one does. A person does things for the sake of accomplishing something. Money generally follows.

— Colonel Henry Crown, owner of the Empire State Building, *The New York Times*, Feb. 21, 1960.

A story about the significance of security was told by Lester L. Coleman, syndicated newspaper columnist and attending surgeon at the Manhattan Eye, Ear and Throat Hospital in New York City. He described his patient Joe, who volunteered for three years of active duty aboard a minesweeper sailing the North Atlantic. It was a particularly hazardous assignment during World War II.

Joe was forced to wear a life jacket on board ship at all times—when eating, sleeping, working, and even into the shower. To Joe, as the months wore on, the life jacket came to represent not the security it should have been, but a target for his repressed hostility toward the surrounding German mines. Even amidst the dangers which he and his shipmates faced daily, getting rid of the life jacket became an overriding goal.

Coleman explained Joe's fixation on the life jacket as the symbol of his insecurity. Coleman said, "To some, the quintessence of security is the simple absence of anxiety. To others, it may be freedom from apprehension or liberation from danger."[1]

The day the war in Europe was declared over, the personnel on Joe's ship dropped the formality and order that usually reigned and shouted with jubilation. Sailors embraced one another in unrestrained joy. In a moment of compulsiveness, Joe, cheered on by his crew mates, suddenly ripped off his life jacket and threw it into the sea.

It bobbed on the surface for only a few seconds; then, the life jacket sank from sight. It possessed no flotation at all. For three years Joe had worn with discomfort this symbol of supposed security, and in reality the life jacket was defective. It just sank!

That is the way it is for a lot of physicians. For them, financial security represents freedom from the dangers of an apprehensive retirement.

Most physicians show their need to feel financially secure by an incessant drive to accumulate more patients and take in more dollars. What they fail to realize is that the dollar volume and patient quantity are not the ultimate source of security. The bottom line is what counts—how much the doctor gets to keep from what he earns.

HOW MUCH SHOULD YOU — OR ANYONE ELSE — EARN?

There's an old joke about the doctor who was disgruntled over the size of the plumber's repair bill for work done.

"I can't get fees like that from the practice of medicine," said the physician.

"I couldn't either," the plumber replied, "and that's why I quit medicine."

Jokes aside, we cannot deny that medical consumers accuse physicians of being plutocrats who keep raising their fees because nobody stops them.

Case in Point: "Sure, I probably earn more than most Americans," replies Robert J. Michtom of Rockville Centre, New York, in medical practice since 1949. He is staff physician at Long Island Jewish Medical Center, South Nassau Communities Hospital and Mercy Hospital, and he is associate professor of clinical medicine at Stony Brook, all on Long Island. In answer to consumer critics, Michtom says, "But one reason I make more money is because I work many more hours. The average work week in the U.S. is now less than 40 hours; some occupations are down to thirty-five. I put in between sixty and seventy hours a week at the office, in the hospital and at medical schools where I teach.

"There's something else," says Michtom. "Except for limited times when colleagues cover for me, I'm constantly on call. My wife gives a dinner party and I have to leave just as the guests arrive. Mealtimes at home are frequently interrupted. My family is used to being left alone evenings and many weekends.

"And don't forget, I don't get overtime pay, sick pay, weekend pay, paid vacations, or many other fringe benefits most salaried workers receive. I have to set up my own retirement plan. As an independent, I pay my full Social Security tax—not half, like a working man. I'm not saying this lowers a typical physician's income to that of the average person. But it does cut down somewhat on those vast riches we're supposed to be accumulating."[2]

How much money a doctor—or anyone else—earns will depend upon his entrepreneurial skill as a businessperson.

In our system of medical care delivery there is room for the physician who is convinced that his combined medical knowledge and business abilities merit a higher income. Also, most private physicians do not lack for business even when there are hard times for everyone else. The result of a 1975 survey by the American Medical Association's *American Medical News* was summarized in the headline, "Recession's Effect on Practice is Slight, Physicians Agree."

Rather than decide for yourself how much money you should earn, three factors are doing it for you.

First, the continued high level of business in health care results from a biological fact: Human beings at all economic levels get sick and need treatment.

Second, much of American medicine has to do with comfort, reassurance and convenience—checkups for healthy babies and other preventive measures—rather than the drama of life-saving surgery or the desperation of an ill-nourished populace.

Finally, "third party payers"—the Government and private health insurance companies—pay $9 out of each $10 charged for hospital care.[3]

The health care industry affects the economic fortunes of every part of the economy and virtually every business of any significant size. It provides a $210 billion volume of business in the United States, and you are one of the industry bosses.

DO YOU KEEP THE FULLEST PERCENTAGE AFTER YOU EARN IT?

Physicians' fees are rising an average of 1½ percent per month across the country, which rides ahead of the current national annual inflation rate. This allows physicians to keep the fullest percentage of income after they earn it. Are you doing the same?

Case in Point: Like most physicians practicing in Chicago and its suburbs, for instance, Howard Traisman and his partner Thomas Marr have found in the last few years that the costs of maintaining and staffing the reception room, the seven examining rooms, and the small laboratory in which they treat their pediatric patients have risen by at least 10 percent.

"We believe that doctors working in our type of treatment setup have to make 50 percent profit, or it just isn't worthwhile," said Traisman, a trim, graying man who moves and talks with cheerful briskness.

Traisman began practicing in 1951, in partnership with his late father, after graduating from Northwestern University's Medical School and completing his pediatric training. His operating costs then took about 35 percent of the fees that he and his father charged.

For the last few years, these costs have risen to 45 percent of their fees, leaving Traisman and Marr 5 percent for contingencies. "I'm getting older every day, I keep getting up just as early as ever, but like a lot of people these days, I'm really not making any more money," Traisman said.

The salaries of the two laboratory technicians, the two receptionists, the secretary-bookkeeper and the cleaning woman that the two pediatricians employ are the biggest factor in their rising operating expenses.

"We've had only a very small increase in the costs of the drugs we administer and we've pretty much held our charges for laboratory tests and shots," Traisman said. However, the rent he pays for his office complex has jumped in the last two years. So have other operating expenses such as postal rates on the 2,000 statements his office mails out each month. The increasing number of insurance and medical forms that his middle-income patients need to have completed adds at least five hours of clerical time to his weekly costs.

"And more than 30 percent of our fees are paid to us on a time basis on credit so to speak, and we don't make any financing charges," advised Traisman. "And collections are certainly getting slower as the weeks go by."[4]

WHY YOU MAY NOT KEEP MUCH OF WHAT YOU EARN

One reason why you appear to need and want financial advice from magazines like *Medical Economics,* which began in October, 1923 and bills itself as "The Business Magazine of the Medical Profession," is that, like professional athletes and movie stars, you are in a high-income group that is incongruously naive about money.

When a businessperson becomes rich, he usually does so by being knowledgeable in his profession, which is business. This means that he automatically knows all about interest rates, investments, management techniques, and other matters that deal with finances. You become rich because you are a noted surgeon, or because you have become a leader in your field of medicine, or because you are in a very rare specialty. You have spent your time and attention studying the human organism's physiology and pathology and not the way it does business.

At the same time, your office may be chaotic and run with a lack of coordinating management in practice. Your billing system may be haphazard, collection ratios abysmal, your personnel may be stealing you blind, overhead costs may be excessive, inventory of medical supplies may be out of control, and your time may be wasted by irrelevant trivia. This poor management may be only the tip of the iceberg that is disregarded by you because you are so immersed in the practice of the art and science of medicine. You may be the so-called "ivory-tower doctor." On the other hand, you may be earning so much money, you have convinced yourself that a little mismanagement does not disturb you.

Money management naiveté makes an "ivory-tower" physician a notoriously easy mark for unscrupulous lawyers and other business people who try to promote a sharp deal. Doctors invest in feed-lot cattle, professional baseball and football teams, experimental motion pictures, exotic resorts, and other glamorous areas that let them "swing a little."

"Sometimes the riskier or crazier the venture, the more appeal it seems to have for them," said a Los Angeles legal secretary who works for two attorneys. She said, "The law partners' main preoccupation is dreaming up phony corporations and thinking up schemes to get doctors to invest in them. None of these corporations ever succeed, but the doctors are suckers and eager to invest. Their contributions range from $2,000 to $25,000 and $50,000. Doctors who complain about getting a return on their investment are quickly bought out. The others just dangle. Doctors understand that all patients do not live after surgery, and they seem to take a similar view when a company in which they've invested fails. They are without a doubt the most vulnerable group of investors in the world."[5]

THE BRIGHT FUTURE FOR INCORPORATED PROFESSIONALS

Luckily, such unscrupulous lawyers are few. The majority make it their business to look out for the best interest of their physician clients. Many lawyers argue that incorporation has done much to lessen financial hazards for physicians. Lawyers maintain that safeguards can be written into incorporation papers even to prevent foolish investments.

The bright future for incorporated professionals involves them in a series of agreements that contain checks and balances. A group of doctors that has formed a corporation, for instance, will have pension funds that amount to several hundred thousand dollars. This kind of money could easily be squandered on fly-by-night investments if left in the hands of a single speculation-prone physician.

Instead, the corporation usually will have retained an investment firm to manage the funds for them. Real estate should never be invested in by the fund. However, investments may be made in mortgages secured by real estate.

Pension funds will not be taxed until a physician begins to draw on them at retirement; or the corporation may put its earnings into a profit-sharing fund where the tax-sheltered money can be invested in a variety of ventures and will eventually be taxed when disbursed as capital. The same tax treatment is given for a pension fund or profit-sharing fund.

As described in Chapter Six, the corporation owns the fixed assets of the physicians' practices, pays for their malpractice insurance and other business expenses, and puts them and other members of the staff on a fixed salary. Sometimes it pays for life and medical insurance for corporate members, although it must then offer comparable plans to the corporation's other employees. Incorporated practices can also provide workmen's compensation plans in case of prolonged illness or injury on the job.

Incorporating has done much to lessen other practice dangers as well—partnerships, for example. Rather than dissolving a partnership, a doctor who disagrees with his colleagues need merely sell his shares in the corporation to another doctor. Thus, "medical divorces" are made easier by incorporation.

PRACTICE PHILOSOPHY DETERMINES YOUR LIFE STYLE

How much you (or anyone else) can earn will depend upon one's philosophy and goals. Is happiness measured in terms of accumulated wealth or in fulfillment of long-range plans for educating the children? Do you feel most secure from knowing there is a substantial retirement program in your future, or from bringing home immediate luxuries such as arrangements for exotic vacations or furs and jewelry?

Planning for the future or living life to its fullest right now are two different things. They are philosophies at variance. With future plans and retirement most paramount, you will set your sights on what growth the practice will require to accommodate those plans. Living up to the hilt immediately is more of a temptation, we admit, and generally has its foundation planted during those lean years when you sacrificed considerably while attending medical school. Enjoying a swinging life style now calls for living on anticipated income.

> *Case in Point:* We recently worked with a physician who was near bankruptcy even while he cleared $126,000 a year. He lived well beyond his means and lost control of his expenses and what he had to earn to pay them.
>
> Franklin Signer of Decatur, Illinois, was audited by the Internal Revenue Service for 1977 and 1978 and received a revised tax bill for $68,500 along with a statement that he signed saying that he agreed with the Government's assessment. Without a penny in the bank to fall back on, Signer was completely unable to pay the bill. He had already borrowed up to the limit that his bankers would allow. Signer was frantic and became ill from his troubles. He had to stop work even though his fixed overhead expenses continued for a whole year.

Formulate Your Family and Practice Budgets and Stick to Them

The solution to Signer's problem, once he returned to practice and found a way to pay off the Government in installments, was to formulate a family budget and an office budget and stick to both of them.

There are essentially two ways of looking at family and practice budgets. One is to consider planned spending with the practiced eye of a watchdog. Watch and evaluate every economic move before you make it. Admittedly, this takes much from the pleasure of living and becomes a wrist-slapping form of exercise.

Another more pleasant way to live within a budget is to look at it with an attitude of growth; use income to maximum advantage. We advise that you make classifications such as payments for insurance, household items, office items, food, clothing, automobile upkeep, utilities, recreation, furniture, education and retirement.

The budget idea is not difficult to establish. Look to your spending in times past and not what has been foolish and what has been needed. Characterize your various expenditures and classify them as to whether or not they were planned and saved for or made on a crisis basis.

In formulating an office budget, we think you should keep informed as to the current costs, consumption rates, and necessary reorder times for medical supplies. This will be done by your responsible personnel who, incidentally, are usually builders of a practice and not contributors to waste.

LET A BANK AUTOMATE YOUR FINANCIAL RECORDS

To increase practice income and decrease office expense, you should be aware of and make use of the benefits afforded by a variety of bank services. Few people do. For example, banks will keep records for you.

Banks tend more and more to support the small businessperson in the security of his business, and yours is considered a small business with services to sell.

Here are some of the bank services your office personnel may put to good use:

- You deposit all cash and check receipts daily into your office savings account. Most banks will transfer savings funds as you request in required amounts into your checking account as you need them for paying bills.
- Some banks will list cancelled checks in the chronological order that your assistant writes them rather than in the order in which the bank receives them. This makes the task of reconciling the bank statement much easier.
- Some banks will categorize expenses for your office through codings on the bank statement. In effect, this is a type of financial statement.
- Most banks will educate you and/or your staff as to the reconciling process.
- Many banks will assume further responsibility for preparing your payroll checks and maintaining the corresponding records. Keeping your payroll money in the bank is all that is required.
- Many banks are set up to handle retirement funds either of the self-employed Keogh plan type or of the corporate program type.
- Some banks execute government reports for pension plans and include accountings of individuals covered in the plan.

THE PAYOFF OF EXPENSE SHARING

Physicians in similar specialties, especially a surgical practice, frequently find advantages in sharing expenses. It is not unusual to find yourself with office space and personnel not fully utilized during an eight-hour workday. You could reasonably sublet the space and share the salaries of employees with another physician. They would be paid in proportion to the time and usage by both doctors. The same could be done with purchasing supplies and equipment.

Some of the specific advantages of expense-sharing most frequently claimed by those who do it are:

• The ability to acquire and use better available equipment for diagnosis and therapy research and for administrative functions.

• The opportunity to enter into practice with less of a heavy professional investment.

• The ease of accessible consultation. You need only wait for your expense-sharing colleague to arrive at the office.

• The ready accessibility of a fellow physician to cover for you right on your own premises, while you attend professional meetings, educational courses or go on vacation.

• The many benefits of group practice without the obvious disadvantages of the direct monetary relationship in sharing income as well. You may keep all that you earn.

ADOPTING THE SUCCESS PHILOSOPHY OF MAXWELL MALTZ

The author of the best-selling book, *Psycho-Cybernetics,* plastic surgeon Maxwell Maltz, used the following acronym to illustrate how you get SUCCESS:

- S – *Sense of direction.* Know where you are heading and the direction others are taking also.
- U – *Understanding.* Realize what your personal needs are and what other persons want as well.
- C – *Courage.* Find courage to be honest with yourself and to be honest when interacting with somebody else.
- C – *Compassion.* Charity, kindness and sympathy are actions you naturally would offer to others but reserve them for yourself too, even though you have made mistakes in the past.
- E – *Esteem.* Before you will ever find happiness, you must feel a personal respect for who you are.
- S – *Self-acceptance.* Accept yourself for what you are and what you have done, not blindly or with false pride but with appreciation.
- S – *Self-confidence.* Setbacks can hold no obstacle to the achievement of your ultimate goals. Feel confident because you have laid out long-term plans steadily and faithfully. Then you will feel even greater self-confidence.

Three Keys to Unlock a Profitable Practice

A distillation of Maxwell Maltz's concepts is stated by his words: "Your days are full of goals. You work to strengthen your internal resources, the success instincts . . ."[6]

Thus he suggests that there are three keys to a profitable practice. They constantly reactivate your success mechanism, which is your built-in capacity to achieve fulfillment.

• The *first key* steers your mind and your every action in the direction of your destiny. It is to *sincerely and enthusiastically set goals.* It has you define your goals and then study the cause and effect relationship of obtaining them.

The single most important business diagnosis you can make is to be sure of what you really want. Knowing that, you will subconsciously provide yourself with a certain power. You feel such a strong desire to get what you want that you are able to achieve over any odds. We call that goal-setting desire "want power." Want power will open doors that might ordinarily be closed to you simply because there is no greater force in your personal world than the power of what you most want.

• The *next key* offers medical practice profitability. It is *the joy that comes with productive work.*

To feel daily, even hourly, the exultation of a person who pours his most productive powers into his work, is the height of contentment. That contentment affords you the ability to work more effectively and approach final goal fruition from the seeds you have planted. Here is where laboratory training, exposure to many clinical patients, hard study, much reading, and many dollars spent bring you the big payoff each day.

The Scottish essayist-historian Thomas Carlyle wrote: "Blessed is he who has found his work; let him ask no other blessedness . . . Even in the meanest sorts of Labor, the whole soul of man is composed into a kind of real harmony the instant he sets himself to work."

• A *third key* for unlocking a profitable practice is to have *realistic expectations of what your want power will permit.*

You cannot fly to the moon without some kind of rocketed missile, or drop to the deepest depths of the sea without a manned small submersible. So it is with goals. Being satisfied with setting them and feeling motivation to attain them are not enough.

> *Case in Point:* A weight-conscious patient, for example, may set a goal to lose twenty-seven pounds in twenty-seven days. It is unlikely that the patient will be able to accomplish this task without a conscientious program of fasting. The expectation is unrealistic even then, if fasting is done merely by instituting the technique of total starvation. The patient will probably hurt himself. He is best served if he takes the time to prepare, in advance, a studious plan of how one must go about losing weight without causing harm to body and mind. His weight loss desire and goal achievement are probably best served if the patient programs himself under a physician's care.

So, too, is your situation of long-term goal planning. You can set the stage on your own, make a decision to grow in practice, then prepare yourself by reading books such as this one. Accomplishment of the task may best be done by then calling for help from a skilled person for an in-depth evaluation of the feasibility of your goals.

In addition, you have to confront and conquer the "I can't" copout. An important consideration is to admit that "I can't" really means "I won't." Once you accept this truth you will begin to build confidence for achieving a skyrocketing net income. Turn the "I can't-won't" mentality into "I will!"

REFERENCES FOR CHAPTER TEN

1. Coleman, Lester. "The significance of security." *Physician's World* 11:3, December 1974.

2. David, Lester. "A physician answers his critics." *Physician's World* 11:29–33, December 1974.

3. Schwartz, Harry. "The health business: built in stability." *The New York Times,* March 30, 1974.

4. King, Seth S. "How a doctor copes: his fees rise with expenses." *The New York Times,* March 21, 1975.

5. Johnson, Sheila K. "My doctor, the corporation." *The New York Times Magazine,* December 29, 1975.

6. Maltz, Maxwell. *Creative Living for Today.* New York: Pocket Books, 1970.

chapter eleven

How to Get Your Personal Finances in Step With This Six-Figure Target

I never met a rich man who was happy, but I have only very occasionally met a poor man who did not want to become a rich man.

— Malcolm Muggeridge, *The New York Times*, April 24, 1978

At the end of each year when sufficient information has been accumulated, you have an obligation to yourself to construct a personal statement of net worth.

Once completed, this statement can be used to measure your progress financially against last year's statement. Check your comparison and ask yourself the following questions:

- Were there marked variations in personal worth?
- What unusual circumstances might explain the changes?
- Did you expect the net effect?
- Did the goals you set last year materialize?

Now, set new goals for the current year. Focus overall on increasing net worth by retiring debts and providing for impending liabilities.

Through analyzing your personal statement and setting future goals, there will be fewer disappointments when you check your net worth next year. You'll have fiscal awareness from planning and review. There will be no misunderstandings.

All too often, a doctor is baffled by whether or not he can afford to purchase a luxury. He may be earning a substantial income, but he wonders how much is being kept. The family balance sheet will let you know exactly how much you have. Greater peace of mind comes from knowing where you are financially.

The balance sheet is an inventory of all assets and liabilities at a given moment. The balance sheet for an individual is the personal statement—a balance of assets and liabilities. All of us hope our assets outweigh our liabilities.

INTERPRETATION OF THE PERSONAL STATEMENT

Family financial management can be developed from putting your personal finances in perspective. Do this by interpreting your assets and liabilities listed on the personal statement.

Lets look at *assets* first:

- *Cash on hand and in banks* – This is an aggregate of all money in regular savings accounts, regular checking accounts, your spouse's savings accounts, certificates of deposit you own.
- *U.S. Government securities* – Limited to Federal Securities, Government bonds, Treasury notes.
- *Listed securities* – Those listed on the stock market as opposed to retained earnings of an unlisted corporation in which you hold an interest.
- *Accounts receivable* – a comfortable discount factor for bad debts is 20 percent of the total of receivables.
- *Real estate owned* – Include the value of the residence you own; especially take note of its market value. Acknowledge the mortgage owed. List the market value of your medical office building, if owned. Show privately owned investment property. A debt on the property would be shown on the liability side of the personal statement.
- *Real estate mortgages receivable* – In the event of sale of a property and taking back a second mortgage or even a first mortgage, this would be a listable asset.
- *Automobiles and other personal property* – The true current market value and not an emotional value is needed.
- *Other assets* – Include pension plans, profit-sharing plans with vested interests, a self-employed Keogh plan even if frozen at an earlier date, additional joint venture assets, limited partnership investments, municipal bonds, and other items.

Tally these assets for an overall picture of positive value.

Liabilities

On the liability side, list all the notes payable that are secured or unsecured, accounts and bills due, unpaid income tax liability, and other items. Note that this personal statement gives an instantaneous picture of your net worth as of December 31 of any given year.

Unpaid tax installments, which normally fall due on January 15th or the balance due on April 15th of the succeeding year, should be listed as a liability. Enter mortgages owed along with other debts. Include loans on life insurance policies.

Composition of Capital

The difference between the assets and liabilities is a figure to be entered as net worth. The size of net worth is important but even more imperative is its composition—capital producing versus capital draining.

The so-called luxury assets such as a second home, an investment in yachts, fancy cars and that sort of thing, are assets that drain. Ask yourself if these items are too heavily nonliquid. Are they too demanding of the cash flow in any crisis situation?

Having your personal statement laid out before you, you can now more readily make decisions.

Asset ownership might be adjusted. For example, you may have too heavy a cash position in banks. Tax shelter investments might be better. Perhaps for more conservative action the purchase of municipal bonds for tax-exempt income is best. Investments for tax spinoffs should be considered, too. The most common spinoffs are found in the real estate market—a tangible and depreciable asset—income-generating but useful in tax strategy deductions.

In one glance you are able to see the total ownership and make decisions regarding assets from perusing the personal statement.

Real estate which has outserved its usefulness may be disposed of. You may decide to take advantage of equity buildup brought about by inflation. The transfer of assets to children and to your spouse for state tax purposes can be decided once your personal finances are in perspective.

Your determination to balance out capital gains against capital losses may be accomplished by seeing exactly where your finances are at any given moment.

The bank or other creditor will usually ask for a net worth statement once a year. You need do it just once and photocopy necessary repeat statements from year to year, unless you make big changes.

In summary, your net worth is the total of everything you own less the sum of everything you owe. If you become aware of where you are financially and where you are going, using the available instruments, the practice of medicine should become more relaxed and effective for you. The personal statement is one of these instruments. It should be made available to your investment counselor, management consultant, attorney, insurance consultant, or others involved with your personal finances.

ESTATE PLANNING

Professional advisors will serve you strictly at your own discretion. In no instance can any single advisor serve the roles of all the professions. It would be dangerous to assume that one individual could perform all the required tasks in estate planning. One professional needs the next.

Too often, an advisor feels that he or she is being encroached upon in his area of expertise, but each advisor should be open-minded concerning another's suggestions. In evaluating your estate planning team, be sure personal jealousies won't interfere with your own best interests.

Legal Advice

The key draftsman of documents necessary in the formation of estate planning is your attorney. His job is to become thoroughly familiar with your estate planning objectives. He will go on to serve as the liaison in directing the total process of estate planning and coordinate matters with other team members. In the probate and postprobate periods, an attorney becomes as vital as he is in the planning stage.

After your death, the attorney has the major duty to implement the estate plan including probate of the will, functioning of trust agreements, the performance of business agreements, and more. He also serves in the extremely important role as constant personal and legal advisor for family members. Consultation between your spouse and your competent family attorney will eliminate most of the problems that will surface during a probate or post probate period.

Management Advice

The management consultant is an essential member of the estate planning team. He or she assists with the accumulation of basic financial data which is critical for estate planning matters and the business affairs of the practice. This advisor holds a strategic position for assisting in the probate and post probate periods. The consultant works with the accountant on accounting forecasts and estate taxation.

Investment Advice

Investment counselors in real estate and securities provide sophisticated and individualized recommendations. They advise on investments for living and for estate planning. Many such counseling firms render a detailed analysis of your investments. Then they tailor an investment program to meet the needs of your living estate including income requirements and capital investing.

Insurance Advice

The insurance advisor is a vital team member, since insurance is essential to life and estate planning. Life insurance, in fact, possesses an unequalled capacity to solve many estate problems. Its proceeds are generally free from income taxation and can be arranged to relieve debt taxes or serve as a family readjustment fund. Life insurance may provide educational funds, keep a family business operating, finance business liquidations or stock retirement agreements, and serve many other needs.

Advice on Trusts

The bank trust officer should be recognized as an estate planning team member. Bank personnel often develop valuable knowledge of your business activities and your personal objectives. They will have special training in estate planning including the problems, solutions, taxation concepts, and other matters. Trust departments offer a wide range of services for you during your lifetime and for your family after your demise.

The trust officer's advice is based not only on prior experience with your objectives but also on his unique ability and expertise in varieties of estate planning and family financial security. Trusts may be used in many effective ways to solve serious estate planning problems. These might include management of assets, providing for one's family care and maintenance, meeting emergency needs such as extended illness, satisfying educational goals, saving income, and saving estate taxes. Trust departments actually specialize in helping families after an untimely death.

The combination of a trust department's special knowledge and the bank's experience with your financial affairs makes the trust officer one of the most effective members of the estate planning team. Where trust services are required, no advisor is more important than the trust department's manager or your assigned officer.

The trust officer may be made the executor of your estate. In that case, he will assure that the estate's assets are accumulated and protected, proper taxation returns are filed, wills and trusts are handled strictly according to their terms, and he will be an independent administrator helping to avoid family disputes and conflicts. He will manage and invest assets for the trust beneficiaries and will exercise discretion to provide financial integrity and responsibility.

You and your spouse should become well acquainted with members of this advisory team on estate planning. Hold in-depth discussions with them. Understand their services and decide to whom a widow or widower would go in time of need.

NECESSARY STEPS IN ESTATE PLANNING

Establishing a will is the first necessary step in estate planning. The inevitable result of dying without a will is that the state, under its specific state laws of intestacy, decides how the property is to be divided. The disposition of assets will be based neither on your wishes nor on the financial needs or abilities of your heirs but on the intestacy statutes of your legal domicile.

In many states, for instance, one's surviving spouse is entitled to only one-third or one-half of the probated property, with children receiving the remaining portion. Access to the children's share is often saddled with complex procedural requirements, and it may be needed by a parent or guardian to meet child-rearing expenses. Where there are no surviving children or their dependents, the spouse may be surprised to find that the estate is to be shared with other relatives of the deceased such as parents, siblings, and even distant relatives, despite differences in their respective needs. Finally, in the absence of relatives, property goes not to friends or selected charities, but to the state.

Legal, probate, and administrative expenses are also likely to be higher in the absence of a valid will. Without your prior legal directives, the court must appoint an administrator to settle your financial affairs. If you leave minor children, a guardian must be appointed, as well, to look out for their interests. These representatives must be bonded at the expense of the estate, a procedure which could have been eliminated by the provision of a will. A choice that should have been yours will have been left to probate law.

Changes in your personal and financial situation or changes in the state laws affecting estates and taxes make keeping your will up-to-date as important as making it in the first place. If your will is not accepted as valid by the court, your property may be subject to the laws of intestacy as though you had done nothing at all.

Piloting Without Lessons

For you to feel content that your estate planning has been satisfactorily completed because there has been an adequate accumulation and a will written can be compared to buying an airplane. Perhaps you've filled it with gasoline, but then you're assuming that your spouse and children, without piloting lessons, can get in and fly it. Having the airplane and gasoline are important, but they are merely the first step in the complete tour. The second step is to have a pilot trained in performance. The pilot may not know about the intricacies of the motor, but he or she should know where the airport is, how to get the plane off the ground, how to return the plane to the airport, and how to land without doing damage to oneself or the aircraft. The individual must also know where to find a good mechanic, how to recognize and heed danger signals, and the importance of not lending the airplane to others. Finally, there is nothing better than having a good map in critical times.

If you know that your spouse is unable to fly the airplane, make appropriate arrangements to help a little with navigation. Have a navigation plan—the estate plan—guidance necessary and in writing. At least, have it in the form of a letter which is to be reviewed upon the death of the primary provider, probably you. Even a tape recording might be reviewed upon your death. Some means of communication is needed to work in conjunction with your estate planning. It will supplement the will and communicate instructions of a personal nature to family members.

Communicate Clearly

Expressed thoughts won't be considered rigid or binding and may be changed; it is necessary to put them in writing. Always temper your instructions by a careful consideration of the facts and circumstances that could exist at the time the decision has to be made. Use customary language. Don't get involved with legal language.

Begin your communication by identifying the location of the various documents and records having to do with the estate. Describe where you have the will, the securities, the life insurance policies. Name the life insurance agent to contact. Tell about business agreements, pensions, documents, profit-sharing plans, stock purchases, corporate forms, trust agreements, various bank accounts, retirement investments, and who has been assisting in these investments.

Include particular directions on whom to contact for legal services, accounting, life insurance advice, banking, the trust people, brokerage in securities, etc. Indicate how you have segregated assets and who might be contacted to give assistance in this area.

Tell how to dispose of personal belongings in this letter or tape recording.

It's not feasible to restate a will each time a new personal item has been secured; simply make a letter entry.

Thus, while the communication is not intended to be a complete recitation of all thoughts which may be indicated in the last will, it should certainly be an aid to that navigator left to guide your estate.

The key to finding valuable papers is to indicate their location on several photocopied pages. Place these photocopies in each place of safekeeping such as your safe-deposit box, home safe, and other places. Update the record and copies annually.

CREATING AN ESTATE TRUST

From the beginning of your estate planning, regard must be given to the distribution of your life's accumulations. Who shall receive them, in what amounts, and how? The will you make can cause your gifts to be paid outright or to be held in trust.

Whatever you give outright after your death or during your lifetime can be used by the recipient as he or she sees fit. It may be sold, spent, wasted, given away, invested profitably or disastrously, or simply lost. A beneficiary may be industrious, frugal, and wise and still be subjected unhappily to the pressures of relatives and friends. How your distribution will be used, therefore, involves important and far-reaching decisions on your part.

Consider the possibilities inherent in trusts. A trust is created when title to property is transferred to a trustee to be used for the benefit of the designated persons. These are the beneficiaries. The trust agreement spells out how your property is to be managed, who is to receive income or otherwise benefit from it, who is to eventually receive the principal, and more. All this is stipulated in a document that creates the trust.

A great virtue of the trust created under a will is that it may be an extension of yourself into the future. You won't be there, but your trustee will be representing your wishes. Give adequate power to the trustee in order to accomplish what you want done.

If you aren't willing to leave such absolute discretion to your trustee, name somebody whom the trustee may consult, or whose instructions the trustee may accept.

The concept of the trust is one of the most ingenious developments in the history of estate and financial planning. It has flexibility. A trust, for example, can be revocable or irrevocable. It can be created during your lifetime (inter vivos) or at death (testamentarily). The trust may be funded upon its creation or serve as an unfunded vehicle to receive assets at some future time.

You can create a trust which will hold and manage your investments and continue to provide security for your family after your death without any interruptions. You may decide to form a trust for a specific purpose such as the education of your children or grandchildren. There are special trusts you can set up to benefit your favorite educational or charitable organization without jeopardizing your financial security or that of your family.

In short, trusts separate the benefits of property ownership from the burdens that usually accompany the management of property, whether it be cash, securities, bonds, life insurance, real estate, business interests or anything else.

There is a rather practical side to trusts. With careful planning and implementation, they can save many thousands of dollars in federal income and estate taxes, thus providing additional funds for the security of your family.

Two basic trust types are available. A testamentary trust is created by a person in his will and comes into existence only at his death. A living trust, which has seen a great increase in use lately, is created by agreement and becomes effective immediately.

The will is still the basic estate planning instrument, however. Trusts created by a will are still the most common trust vehicle.

Such a testamentary trust furnishes certain benefits:

1. *Family protection.* The desire to provide for the support and education of a spouse and children will best be achieved by means of a trust which authorizes the trustee to utilize both the income and principal for these purposes. From inexperience, naiveté, imprudence, or some other reason, property may be lost by your inheritors in unwise investments. With a testamentary trust, either you or the court will appoint a legal guardian to administer the inheritors' shares, if they are minors. Guardianship proceedings are often burdensome and expensive, but they can be avoided by your use of a trust agreement.

2. *Investment supervision.* By selecting a trustee skilled in handling investments, you can be reasonably assured that your property will be invested prudently under all kinds of economic conditions. It may then serve the best interests of your family.

3. *Tax savings.* Estate tax savings may be achieved not only by taking advantage of the marital deduction allowed, for example, but you can also avoid an unnecessary second tax on your estate. The trust device permits your spouse to enjoy the economic benefits of the property during his or her lifetime without having it included in his or her estate for federal estate tax purposes.

Savings on taxes can also be achieved by avoiding the inclusion of the property in your children's taxable estates. Yet, they may enjoy its benefits for life. Income taxes of your beneficiaries may further be minimized by providing for "spraying" or "sprinkling" of income among members of the family as needed for their support, education, and other purposes.

chapter twelve

How Corporate Pension Plans Help You Reach The Quarter-Million Goal

The retirement income problem in the United States has become a retirement income crisis.

— Senate Special Committee on Aging, "Economics of Aging," January 18, 1971.

Age is only a number, a cipher for the records. A man can't retire his experience. He must use it. Experience achieves more with less energy and time.

— Bernard Baruch, on his 85th birthday, August 20, 1955.

In earning a quarter of a million dollars a year for most of the years you are in practice, the practical problem of how to sock it away for retirement is not an easy one to solve. A solid, cumulative pension plan is mandatory, and the best plan will be established in a professional corporation (P.C.). The question arising is which type of corporate pension plan is correct for you and your P.C.?

To begin with, it is important to understand that the expression "Pension Plan" is a generic term applied to *Defined Benefit* and *Defined Contribution Plans,* as well as *Pension* and *Profit-Sharing Plans.* Further, realize that what we are stating in this chapter is merely a general guide for your review of existing or proposed plans; for detailed assistance, you should consult with members of your advisory team, a management consultant and/or your attorney.

To review the plan, we must first understand *what* we are reviewing. A Defined Benefit type of plan is one which has *retirement benefits* based upon a predetermined formula such as a percentage directly related to average annual compensation. This is commonly known as a Flat Benefit Pension Plan, or it may be figured as compensation per year of service, which is known as a Unit Benefit Pension Plan.

The Defined Contribution Plan prescribes annual levels of contributions to the plan without concern for the amount of benefits that will be available at retirement time; it pays benefits based solely on accumulated amounts. The contribution is related to a percentage of current compensation.

Indeed, there are limitations placed upon each type of plan, but in differing ways. The Defined Benefit Plan limits *retirement* benefits currently to the lesser of $124,500 or 100 percent of the participant's average compensation for the three consecutive years in which his compensation was the highest. The average of the highest five-years compensation may be used if the plan is integrated (more on integration later). Such limitation is adjusted annually to reflect increases in the cost of living. Our best guess is that the present limitation will increase by $10,000 per year from now on. Typically, the Internal Revenue Service submits a news release in mid-February adjusting limitations. Annual contributions may not exceed amounts actuarially necessary to fund a straight life annuity commencing no earlier than age 55 or after 10 years' service with the employer.

Defined Contribution Plans, which include Profit-Sharing and Money Purchase Pension Plans, limit *annual contributions* to an amount equal to 25 percent of direct compensation. A Profit-Sharing Plan standing alone is limited to 15 percent of compensation to employees covered by the plan. Annual contributions are currently limited to $41,500, which is also subject to annual adjustment based on the cost of living index application. This limitation will probably be increased by about $3000–$5000 per year. You should keep in mind that while a Profit-Sharing Plan does not require annual contributions, a Pension Plan does require annual contributions, at the fixed percentage of compensation rate.

A combination of plans may be used in a corporate setting. In any case in which a participant is a participant in both a Defined Benefit Plan and a Defined Contribution Plan maintained by the same employer, the sum of the Defined Benefit fraction and the Defined Contribution fraction may not exceed 1.4.

The Defined Contribution fraction is the result reached from the following fraction:

$$\frac{\text{SUM OF ANNUAL ADDITIONS TO PARTICIPANT'S ACCOUNT AS OF CLOSE OF THE YEAR}}{\text{SUM OF THE MAXIMUM AMOUNT OF ANNUAL ADDITIONS WHICH COULD HAVE BEEN MADE}}$$

As shown, this area is complex and certainly specifics must be reviewed with the assistance of competent advisors.

Generally speaking, the Defined Benefit Plan allows for greater annual contributions than does the Defined Contribution Plan. Although such contributions are deductible, you should give careful consideration to the fixed demands of large contributions. Too often the tax deferral reality interferes with good judgment as relates to a personal cash squeeze analysis. You should bear in mind that mandated contributions can create a problem for an existing standard of living. A doctor must, of course, prepare for retirement but he or she should be reminded that today is as important a day in one's life as the days of retirement. We suspect that the reminder might be the doctor's spouse.

Many times, an anxiety to reduce immediate taxes gets confused with long-range planning. It is logical to presume a fully funded Defined Benefit Retirement Program at age 55, but if this attainment comes through denial of earlier years' comforts, then the judgment may not have been prudent. Also, doctors in joint practices generally have difficulty, since a fellow stockholder may be senior in age with greater annual contributions indicated to a Defined Benefit Plan. Any offsetting adjustments in direct salaries may be challenged by the Internal Revenue Service as a salary reduction program which is forbidden and may threaten the viability of the corporate structure. Under certain circumstances, a corporation's Board of Directors may restrict contributions to be based on varying levels of corporate compensations.

A situation may arise where a Defined Benefit Program becomes fully funded and the Board wishes to continue contributing to a retirement plan. The Defined Benefit Plan may then be "frozen" and a Money Purchase (Defined Contribution) Plan may be activated. There is a limitation as to the size of the plan to be created requiring discussions with advisors at that time.

Now that the basic characteristics of various types of plans have been pointed out, a review of general provisions under the plans is indicated. Our approach here is to indicate requirements and—where applicable—to make recommendations:

QUALIFICATION OF PLANS – Your plan, to qualify, must cover at least 70 percent of all employees, in addition to covering 80 percent of the eligible employees. A plan will not qualify if the Internal Revenue Service finds that it discriminates in favor of officers, shareholders or highly compensated employees.

In addition, corporate officers must be aware that the Internal Revenue Service has been granted authority by both Congress and the Courts to disqualify currently qualified retirement programs if the programs are not maintained in an up-to-date status. In the event that the Internal Revenue Service should issue new Treasury Regulations or should the law in a particular area be changed, it is normal that a corporate retirement plan must be amended to take into account these changes within the year following the year in which such change occurs. In the event that such modification is not made, it is possible that the Internal Revenue Service could then attempt to retroactively disqualify the retirement program. It is therefore imperative that the officers of professional corporations specifically discuss with their professional advisors the need to be informed as to all material changes in the pension area so that plans can be maintained in an up-to-date status.

ELIGIBILITY – Participation must be granted to all full-time employees after one year of service for those employees who have reached the age of twenty-five. However, the one year of service requirement may be extended to three years, if the plan provides for full and immediate vesting of the participant's account balance after the satisfaction of the eligibility period.

A Defined Benefit Plan is permitted to exclude employees who are within five years of normal retirement age at the time they would otherwise become eligible to participate, but only if the exclusion does not result in prohibited discrimination in coverage. Special attention must be given to the percentages rules as indicated above in the *Qualification of Plans*.

A year of service is defined for purposes of determining when an employee is eligible to participate, as a twelve-month period during which the employee performs 1,000 or more hours of work. Participation may not be delayed beyond the earlier of:

(a) The next plan anniversary or,

(b) Six months after completion of the eligibility requirements.

A period of employment prior to a break in service must be aggregated. Credit must be given for this time. However, a plan may require a one-year waiting period before the pre-break and post-break service must be aggregated. Credit is to be given for that year.

Certainly, a long-range perspective is indicated in the review of documenting eligibility standards. Once a plan gains approval from the Internal Revenue Service, it is unwise to consider restrictive changes, as the IRS could challenge and ultimately deny amendments which appear to discriminate in favor of highly compensated individuals.

CONTRIBUTIONS – Caution is once again necessary in deciding on the level of mandated contributions. Pension plans require annual deposits. A delayed contribution for Pension or Profit-Sharing plans may be extended if made within 2 1/2 months after the close of a corporate year. An additional extension may be attained through an extension of filing the corporate income tax return up to an additional six months.

Voluntary participant contributions are permitted, generally to a maximum of 10 percent of the participant's compensation. However, a limit of 6 percent is applied or one-half of such voluntary contribution if the contribution forces the total annual allocation beyond the limitations earlier indicated.

Allocations to participants may be made in accordance with a formula integrating Social Security benefits. For example, a formula may prescribe that 7 percent of excess base compensation shall be allocated to each participant in proportion to the ratio which the excess base compensation bears to the total excess base of all participants. Excess base compensation may be any amount up to the limit of compensation currently set as the maximum compensation used to determine Social Security contributions. Currently this amount is $29,700. A sample of how integrating a plan would work in favor of the principal is illustrated below.

	DR. JONES	AIDE SMITH	AIDE BROWN
PROPORTIONATE % SHARE OF ELIGIBLE SALARIES	80%	10%	10%
SALARIES	$80,000	$10,000	$10,000
INTEGRATION LEVEL	10,000	10,000	10,000
EXCESS BASE COMPENSATION	$70,000	0	0
INTEGRATION FACTOR	.07	.07	.07
COMPUTATION I ALLOCATION	$ 4,900	0	0
COMPUTATION II ALLOCATION	4,080	510	510
TOTAL CONTRIBUTION	$ 8,980	$ 510	$ 510

As you can see, the doctor received benefits of $8,980 which figures as 11.2 percent of salary, while in the aggregate, common law employees received $1,020 or 5.10 percent of salaries, reflecting a reduction of the presumed straight line 10 percent contribution, which otherwise would see $1,000 contributed for each of the aides.

The computations indicated above as "I" and "II" are best viewed as follows:

PRESUMING 10% CONTRIBUTION	$10,000
COMPUTATION I ALLOCATION	4,900
COMPUTATION II ALLOCATION	$ 5,100

After allowing for 7 percent of excess base compensation ($4,900), the remainder amount, $5,100, is apportioned to the eligible employees in accordance with their percentage of total eligible salaries.

SEPARATE ACCOUNT BALANCES – A Defined Contribution Retirement Program requires that each participant's account balance be separately maintained, at least from an accounting standpoint. While this does not necessarily mean that each participant's account must be separated for investment purposes, and it is most common to find that all such account balances are commingled, it is sometimes found to be in the best interests of the plan to allow each participant to retain certain investment discretion over the assets in his or her account. In such circumstances, a participant would have the ability to designate to the trustee the type of assets or specific assets, under certain circumstances, to be invested in by the trustee on behalf of such participant. Under such circumstances, the gains or losses of the participant would be charged directly against such participant's account.

TERMINATION OF PARTICIPATION – Generally speaking, participation in a fund will cease upon the following conditions:

1. Retirement,
2. Termination of employment,
3. Total and permanent disability,
4. Death.

Whereas it is important to specify an age as normal retirement, we believe that a deferred retirement date should be left optional for the corporate directors with participation to continue through the extension of the retirement age.

BENEFICIARIES AND PARTICIPANTS – The plan should allow participants to designate a beneficiary or beneficiaries in case of death. Such designation should include contingent or successive beneficiaries. Notwithstanding the above allowance, specific language should be considered to cover a participant's account in the event no designation was made. Individual state estate statutes should be considered in this regard.

DISTRIBUTIONS – Options must be recited as mediums of payment of benefits. Such options may allow for

1. Cash
2. An Insurance Policy or Insurance Annuity
3. Investments valued at fair market value

The method of payment could allow for:

1. Lump Sum,
2. Annuity Payments,
3. Equal installments over a reasonable period of time.

If an insurance policy is incorporated in the account, then such policy could be transferred or surrendered for cash values. If the payout was activated by death of the participant, then the proceeds of the policy should be paid to the beneficiary. Distributions should be made pursuant to beneficiary directive no later than 60 days after the end of the plan year in which the latest of the following occurs:

1. The participant reaches normal retirement age, or
2. 10 years have elapsed from the time the participant commenced participation in the plan.

At the discretion of the trustee, an earlier payout may be made, presumably taking into consideration any breach of employment agreements, whether or not such payout will be in the best interests of the participant or whether the participant was terminated for misconduct or dishonesty.

VESTING – Generally speaking, the following alternative schedules are acceptable by the Internal Revenue Service for approval of plans. They are:

1. *5–15 year graded vesting.* This schedule requires 25 percent vesting after five years plus 5 percent per year for the next five years of service and 10 percent a year for the subsequent five years, thus resulting in 100 percent vesting after 15 years of service.
2. *Full vesting after 10 years of service.* Since no vesting is granted under this schedule until an employee has completed ten years of service, in high turnover situations, this schedule may prove to be the easiest and perhaps the least expensive to administer.
3. *Modified Rule of 45.* Under this rule, as it is now understood, an employee with at least five years of service and with respect to whom the sum of his age and years of service equals or exceeds forty-five, must be 50 percent vested; for each additional year of service, his interest must vest another 10 percent. In addition, all employees must be 50 percent vested after completing ten years of service, regardless of age, with an accrued vesting

of 10 percent for each year of service thereafter. Service as a nonparticipant prior to age 22 need not be taken into account for vesting purposes.

In actuality, the law provides another alternative, limited to Profit-Sharing Plans; plans can be structured which call for "class year" vesting over not more than five years. Minimum vesting requirements are satisfied for such plans if 100 percent vesting is provided within five years after the end of the plan year for which contributions were made. This has the effect of fully vesting contributions for any given plan year, five years after the date of contribution.

In reality, the vesting schedule quite commonly used by professional corporations is one known as the "committee report schedule." This schedule is not found in ERISA or the Internal Revenue Code, but is found in the Committee Reports adopted by the Joint Committee of Congress. The Committee Reports indicate that normally the following vesting schedule will not be subject to attack by the Internal Revenue Service unless it can be shown that there is a preconceived plan to terminate employees to avoid vesting them under this plan. This schedule is as follows:

NUMBER OF YEARS OF SERVICE	PERCENT VESTED
Less than 4 years of service	0%
4 years but less than 5 years	40%
5 years but less than 6 years	45%
6 years but less than 7 years	50%
7 years but less than 8 years	60%
8 years but less than 9 years	70%
9 years but less than 10 years	80%
10 years but less than 11 years	90%
11 years or more	100%

FORFEITURES – Subject to the provisions of the vesting schedule, forfeitures may occur from time to time. The plan or plans should specifically indicate treatment of such forfeitures; for instance, these amounts would be applied to reduce subsequent contributions under the plan. There is no requirement to reinstate forfeited amounts if a terminated employee is rehired.

PARTICIPANT LOANS – A plan may lend assets to participants if such loans are available to all participants and beneficiaries on a reasonably equal basis, are not made available to highly compensated employees, officers or shareholders in amounts greater than available to other employees, bear reasonable rates of interest and are adequately secured. It is important to establish a repayment schedule with interest charged at a rate not less than the then "prime rate."

PORTABILITY – In the eventuality that an employee might terminate employment and wish a tax-free rollover of vested interest in a subsequent employer's plan, a provision to accommodate such portability should be contemplated. The provision must require that any subsequent employer have a qualified plan, with an indemnification to the transferring corporation accepted by the employee.

In reviewing the elements of this chapter you should realize that this presentation is neither detailed nor definitive and is only intended as a general guide in a review of existing or proposed plans. The ultimate design of a retirement program is one where expertise and experience is critically indicated. Don't leave the area of plan design to amateurs.

Index

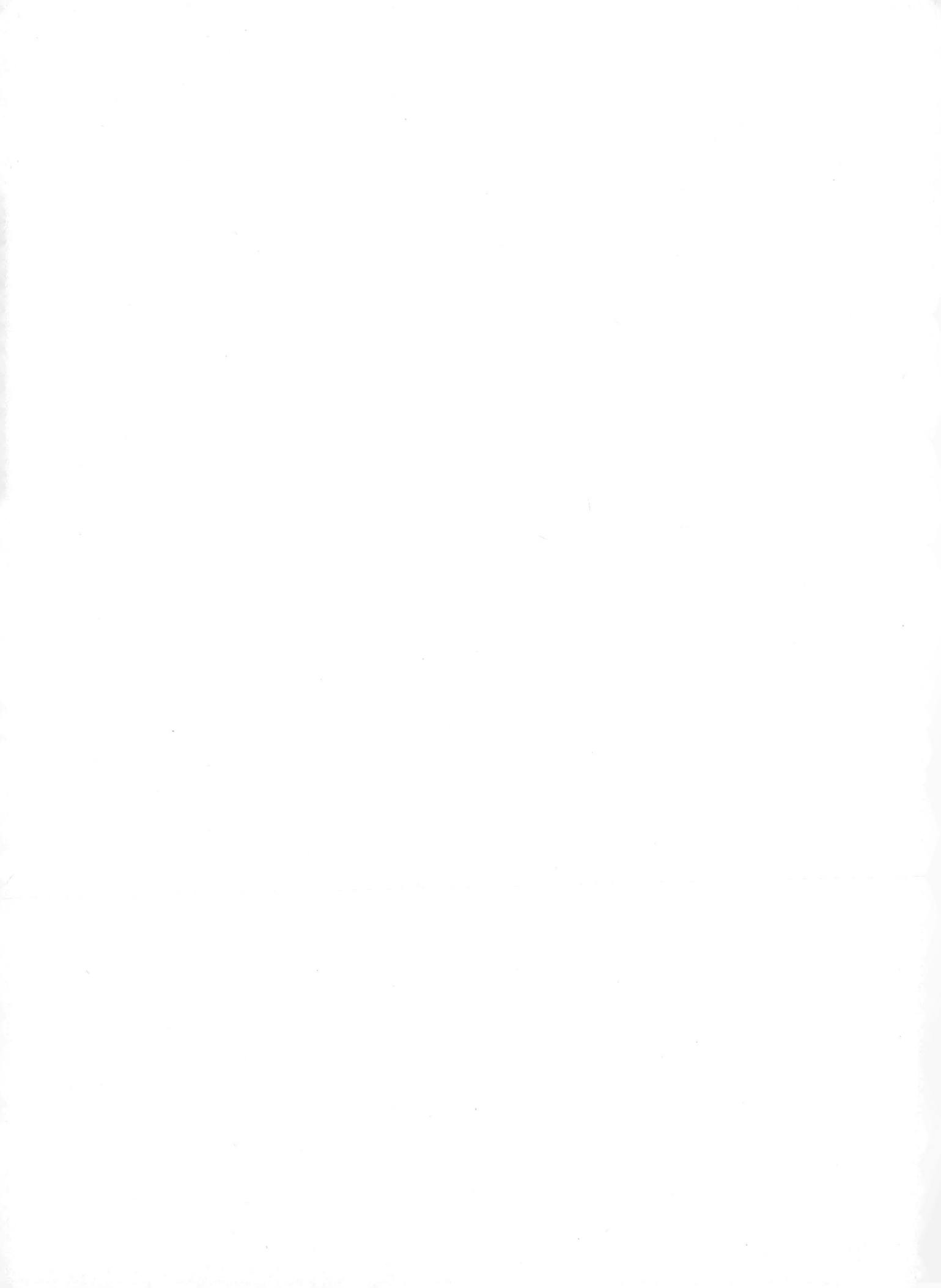

A

Acceptance by medical community, 51–52
Accounts receivable control (*see* Office procedures: practice income)
Advertising, professional, 54–55
Albert Einstein College of Medicine, 88
Amatono, Louis, 63
American Arbitration Association, 71
American Association of Medical Clinics, 86
American Board of Arbitration, 86
American College of Radiology, 21
American Medical Association, ten ethical principles of, 50–51
American Medical Association (*see* Office policy)
American Medical News, 170
American Rehabilitation Foundation, 87
Ankerholz, Donald L., 139, 140
Anxiety-ridden patient: guidelines for evaluation, 66–67
Appley, Lawrence, 109
Application for employment (*figure*), 123–127
Appointments, scheduling, 114
Arbitration (*see* Malpractice: claims)
Ardell, Donald B., 59
Art of Professional Practice Management, The, 11
Associated Credit Men of New York, 160
Attitude, effect on practice growth, 55–56
Audit, medical practice (*see* Medical practice audit)
Automation of financial records (*see* Income)
Auxiliary patient care facilities (*see* Management: twelve strategic approaches)

B

Bank services (*see* Income)
Barrett, Charles, 84
Baruch, Bernard, 189

Belli, Melvin M., 70
Belsky, Marvin S., M.D., 37–39
    Patient-Physician Feedback Group, 37–38
Beneficiaries and participants (*see* Pension plans)
Benefits of estate trusts (*see* Estate trusts)
Blue Cross, 97
Blue Shield, 97
Blum, Richard H., 64
Brawley v. Heymann, 64
Budgeting (*see* Income)
Bunker, John P., 88
Burns, H.S.M., 137
Business manager, 29–32
    fourteen daily audits of, 30–32

C

Carlyle, Thomas, 177
Carter, Alvin, 54
Cayman Islands, 9
Charge slip (*illustration*), 31
Charge ticket (*see* Fees)
Chinese laundry, running practice like, 57
Coleman, Lester L., 169
Collection agency (*see* Fees)
Collection letters (*see* Fees)
Collections, 11
Commission on Medical Malpractice, 1974, 64
"Committee work," time budget chart, 119
Community credit bureau (*see* Fees: patient credit)
Community work (*see* Management: twelve strategic approaches)
Competition, friendly, in medical practice, 49–50
Consultantship after retirement (*see* Incorporated practice)
Consultation, 11–12

Contract buying (*see* Office staff: inventory system)
"Controlled accuracy" (*see* Office procedures)
Control-o-fax, 134
Corporate medicine:
  motivations for joining, 78
Corporation:
  (*see* Incorporated practice)
  definition, 95
  pension fund, 173
  pure, six characteristics of, 96
  reasons for, 95
Cotton, Horace, 52
Council on Medical Service of the American Medical Association, 86
Country doctor, 79–80
  bill collections, 79–80
Crane, Charles A., 160
Crane, G. W., 42
Crimpgraf colors (*see* Office staff: inventory control)
Crown, Henry, 167

D

Daily log (*see* Office procedures: practice income)
Davis, Joseph, 84
Deadbeats, 159–160
  nine danger signals of, 159–160
Defensive medicine, menace of practicing (*see* Malpractice: claims)
Defined Benefit plan (*see* Pension plans)
Defined Contribution plan (*see* Pension plans)
Delegating authority (*see* Office staff)
Detail men (*see* Physician, tips for saving time)
Disability insurance premiums, 97

E

Earnings (*see* Income)
Economic Recovery Act of 1981, 102
"Economics of Aging," 189
Edison, Thomas A., 147
Ekblom, John, 93
Ellwood, Paul M., 87
Emerson, Ralph Waldo, 44
Employee grievances (*see* Physician, tips for saving time)
Employee Performance Appraisal (*figure*), 130

Employer policy manual, 128–129
Employee Retirement Income Security Act:
  establishment of, 96
  functions of, 96
ERISA (*see* Employee Retirement Income Security Act)
Estate planning:
  advice on trusts, 184–185
  communication, 186–187
  insurance advice, 184
  investment advice, 184
  legal advice, 183–184
  management advice, 184
  necessary steps, 185–187
  like piloting without lessons, 186
  will, 185
Estate trusts, 187–188
  benefits, 188
    family protection, 188
    investment supervision, 188
    tax savings, 188
Ethical principles, ten, for making money, 50–51
Ethical ways of getting known, six, 53–55
Evening evaluation (*see* Personal relations technique)
Expense sharing (*see* Income)

F

Factoring (*see* Fees)
Family balance sheet (*see* Personal finances)
Family protection (*see* Estate trusts)
Fang, Bartholomew Bruce, 54
"Fedicare," 12
Fee adjustment, 34
Feedback (*see* Patient feedback)
Fees:
  battle over, 155–156
  best billing procedure, 161–162
  charging by the minute, 152
  charge ticket, 152–153
  collection letters, 162–163
  collections, 155–156
  cyclical billing, 161
    computerized, 161
    manual, 161
  explaining charges, 153–154
  factoring, 166
  finance charges, 156
  follow-up on delinquent accounts, 163–164

INDEX

Fees *(cont'd)*
  legal action, 165
  office policy on business matters, 157
  patient credit:
    application, 157–159
    bureau, 158–159
    capacity, 151
    capital, 157
    character, 151
    community credit bureau, 158–159
    conditions, 157
    information from, 158
  pay-as-you-go, 160–161
  preference for odd amounts, 151–152
  presentation of, 154
    without guilt, 154–155
  selecting collection agency, 164
Financial goal, 21
Flat Benefit Pension Plan *(see Pension plans)*
Fleming, Samuel, 61
Flintner, Morgan, 21
Ford, Henry, 43
Forfeitures *(see Pension plans)*
Furnishings and equipment *(see Management: twelve strategic approaches)*

G

Gillette, Robert D., 81
Glumby, Walter, 81
Greco, Ray S., 82–83
Group Health Cooperative of Puget Sound, 91
Group life insurance *(see Incorporated practice)*
Group practice:
  benefits for patients, 87–88
  definition, 86
  prepayment type *(see Health Maintenance Organization)*
  ten advantages for physicians, 88–89
  ten disadvantages for physicians, 89
  types of, three, 87
Gunderson, Gunnar, 35

H

Haecox, Maynard L., 115
Hamlin, Clay W., 42
Harney, David M., 71
Harris, Louis, 153

Health care cost cutting, 12
Health insurance premiums, 97
Health Maintenance Organization:
  patient care in, 90
  quality of care, 91
  target area, 90
  using institutional facilities, 91
Health Services Research Center, 87
Hiring procedures *(see Personnel)*
HMO *(see Health Maintenance Organization)*
Horace, 13
Hospital corridor consultation *(see Physician, tips for saving time)*
Hospital rounds *(see Physician, tips for saving time)*
House calls *(see Physician, tips for saving time)*
Human relations, principles for daily practice, 44
  ten commandments of, 43–44

I

Income:
  amount of, 170–171
  automation of financial records, 174–175
  bank services, 174–175
  budgeting, 174
    family, 174
    office, 174
  expense sharing, 175–176
    advantages, 175–176
  keeping fullest percentage, 171–172
  long-term goal planning, 177
  losing earnings, 172
  Maxwell Maltz's concepts, 176–177
    three keys to profitable practice, 176–177
  mismanagement, 172
  and practice philosophy, 173–174
  risky investments, 172
  unscrupulous lawyers, 172, 173
Incorporated practices:
  advantages, 96–97
  attorneys' fees, 100
  changes in office procedure, 100–102
    accounting records, 101
    annual franchise tax, 102
    annual reports with state, 102
    bank account, 101
    borrowing from commercial banks, 102
    calling cards, 101

Incorporated practices *(cont'd)*
    with departments of public aid, 101
    equipment, 101
    income tax returns, 101–102
    insurance policies, 101
    leases, 101
    professional license, 101
    purchase-order forms, 101
    signs and directories, 101
    stationery, 101
    telephone numbers, 100–101
  common questions and answers, 98–99
  consultantship after retirement, 97–98
  cost of formation, 99–100
  deferred compensation benefits, 97
  group life insurance, 98
  reimbursed medical expenses, 97
  social security costs, 100
  taxation exclusion, 98
  when inadvisable, 100
Individual Retirement Account *(see* Self-employed retirement plans)
Insurance advice *(see* Estate planning)
Insurance companies, 27
Internal Revenue Service, 33
Interview for personnel appraisal *(see* Personnel)
Inventory system *(see* Office staff)
Investment supervision *(see* Estate trusts)
Investment advice *(see* Estate planning)
Investments, risky, 172

J

Jackson, Everett, 68
Jaffe, Ernst R., 88
Johnson, Fletcher James, Jr., 49
Joint practice, 83–86
  advantages, 83
  disadvantages, 83
  partners as agents of one another, 84
  secrets of successful, 83–84
  ten vital articles in partnership agreement, 84–86
Jordan, Robert A., 26
Jung, Carl, 66

K

Kaiser Foundation Health Plans, 191
Kaiser Permanente experience, 90

Keogh plan *(see* Self-employed retirement plans)
Kidd, William H., 152
Kimbrow, Alex, 147

L

Ladimer, Irving, 71
Lakein, Alan, 116
Lavine, Leroy, 70
Legal action *(see* Fees)
Legal advice *(see* Estate planning)
Lincoln, Abraham, 61
Loans, participant *(see* Pension plans)
Location *(see* Management: twelve strategic approaches)
Long-term goal planning *(see* Income)

M

Malpractice:
  one of first decisions, 61–62
  and special interest groups, 62
Malpractice claims:
  anxiety-ridden patient *(see* Anxiety-ridden patient)
  arbitration, question of, 71–72
  and dentists, 63
  Medical Malpractice Accident Fund *(see* Medical Malpractice Accident Fund)
  menace of defensive medicine, 70
  prevention of, ten point checklist, 69
  rate of, 62–63
  real reasons for, 68–69
  suit-prone doctors, 64–65
  suit-prone patients, 65–66
  why made, 64
Malpractice premiums in California, 62
Malpractice suits, 11
Maltz, Maxwell, 19, 28, 176
Management advice *(see* Estate planning)
Management, twelve strategic approaches, 22–28
  community work, 28
  furnishings and equipment, 25–26
  location, 23–24
  medical service contracts, 28
  office design, 24–25
  patient relations, 24
  patient perceptions, 24

Management approaches (cont'd)
  professional relations, 27
  saying "thank you," 27–28
  systems and policies, 25
  third party involvements, 27
Management techniques:
  four P's of ideal management, 111–136
    patient (see Patient)
    personnel, supporting (see Personnel, supporting)
    physician (see Physician)
    practice (see Practice management)
Marcus Welby, M.D., 155
Marks, E. Jones, 115
Marmaduke, Austin P., 79
Marr, Thomas, 171
Maugham, Somerset, 149
Mayo Clinic, 87
Medicaid, 22
Medical community, gaining acceptance in, 51–52
"Medical divorces," 173
Medical Economics, 172
Medical group (see Group practice)
Medical Group Management Association, 86
Medical Malpractice Accident Fund:
  working of, 72–73
Medical practice audit, 28–29
  questions to be asked, 29
Medical service contracts (see Management: twelve strategic approaches)
Medicare, 12, 21, 22
Merck, George, 75
Meyerson, Irving, 154
Michtom, Robert J., 170
Money Purchase Pension Plans (see Pension plans)
Muggeridge, Malcolm, 179
Multipart Service-Receipt (see Office procedure)
Murray, Robert K., 140

N

Nennhaus, H. Peter, 34

O

Obstetrical work (see Physician, tips for saving time)
Office design (see Management: twelve stra-

Office design (cont'd)
  tegic approaches)
Office layout and space, 114
Office policy:
  American Medical Association's booklet on, 45–46
Office procedures:
  basic rule, 133
  "controlled accuracy," 133
  machines, 133
  practice income, 133–134
    accounts receivable control, 136
    cash disbursements, 135–136
      filing by month, 135
      three-on-page checkbook, 136
    pegboard system, 134–135
      applications, 134–135
      three copies of multipart service-receipt, 135
    petty cash system, 136
    separate daily log, 133–134
Office staff:
  contract buying, 145
  delegating authority to, 139
    checklist of office tasks, 142–144
    history and patient contact tasks, 141
    laboratory, x-ray, and related tasks, 141–142
    physical examination tasks, 140
    reasons for, 139
    therapy tasks, 140–141
  inventory system, 144–146
    bargains, 145
    control, 145–146
      case study, 146
      Crimpgraf® colors, 146
      equipment needed, 147
      installing, 145–146
      storage limitations, 145
    contract buying, 145
    waste avoidance, 144–145
  members of, 139
  nonproductive office time, 147–148
  waste-preventing actions, eleven, 148
Operating costs, 11

P

Pain, meaning of, 41
Patient:
  process of exit for, 114–115

Patient (cont'd)
   scheduling appointments, 114
   telephone patterns, 112–114
     after hour charges, 113
     answering service, 113
     automatic dialing device, 114
     automatic phone answering machine, 114
     beepers, 113
     code password, 113
     ending calls, 113
     "locker room" time, 112
     log, 112
     pay phone in waiting room, 113
     recalls on unlisted lines, 113
     role of receptionist, 112, 113
     Touch-Tone® telephones, 113
     wall phones, 113
Patient credit application (see Fees)
Patient perceptions (see Management: twelve strategic approaches)
Patient referrals:
   from certain actions, 52–53
   from key patients, 57–58
   thirteen questions to ask, 56–57
Patient feedback:
   obtaining, 39
   thirty benefits from, 39–40
Patient-Physician Feedback Group (see Belsky, Marvin)
Patient relations (see Management: twelve strategic approaches)
"Patients' Bill of Rights," 40
Pegboard system (see Office procedures)
Pension plans:
   beneficiaries and participants, 195–196
   Defined Benefit, 191–193
     Flat Benefit Pension Plan, 191–193
     Unit Benefit Pension Plan, 191–193
   Defined Contribution, 191–193
     Defined Contribution Money Purchase Pension Plans, 192
     Profit Sharing Plans, 192
   eligibility, 193
   forfeitures, 197
   participant loans, 197
   portability, 198
   qualification of, 193
   separate account balances, 195
   termination of participation, 195
   social security benefits, 194–195
   vesting, 196–197
P/E ratio (see Physicians' / Earnings Ratio)

Personal finances:
   assets, 182
     accounts receivable, 182
     cash, 182
     listed securities, 182
     personal property, 182
     real estate, 182
     U.S. government securities, 182
   capital, composition of, 182–183
   estate planning (see Estate planning)
   estate trust (see Estate trust)
   family balance sheet, 181
   liabilities, 182
   personal statement, 181–183
Personality traits, seven basic, 42–43
Personal relations technique, 67–68
   evening evaluation, 67–68
Personal statement (see Personal finances)
Personnel:
   bonus arrangement, 129
   employee policy manual, 128–129
   hiring procedures, 121–128
     credit check, 122
     newspaper ad, 121
     notice on bulletin board, 122
     probationary period, 128
     references, 122
     salary adjustments, 128
     word of mouth, 122
   need for assistant, 120–121
   optional inclusions, 129
     continuing medical education, 129
     duties clearly stated, 129
     patients' confidences, 129
     team approach, 129
   paid vacation time, 129
   part-time employees, 128
   qualifications for aides, 121
   salary review, 128
   sick leave, 129
   tips for actual performance appraisal, 132–133
     concentration on behavior and facts, 132
     positive attitude, 132
     salary discussion, 133
     self-improvement plans, 133
     setting for interview, 132
     specific goals and targets, 133
     timing of interview, 132
     two-way communication, 132
     using satisfactory areas of performance, 132

Personnel *(cont'd)*
  tips for pre-performance appraisal, 129–132
    dismissal, 132
    evaluation policy, 130
    isolating reasons for unsatisfactory work, 132
    study of job behavior, 130
Petty cash system (*see* Office procedures: practice income)
Pharmacist, forms for (*see* Physician, tips for saving time)
Physician's absence, 120
Physician, tips for saving time, 116–118
  aide fielding patients' questions, 118
  bill discussion, 118
  cash payments, 118
  charges for insurance forms, 117
  chart holders, 118
  color coding, 118
  "committee work," 118
  daily planning, 117
  detail men, 117
  dictation procedures, 118
  direct telephone to central dictation, 117
  elimination of hospital corridor consultation, 117
  hobbies and relaxation, 117
  hospital and patient needs, 118
  hospital rounds, 117
  house calls, 117
  moveable equipment, 118
  obstetrical work, 117
  one floor of hospital plan, 117
  one hospital plan, 117
  patient and hospital procedures, 118
  periods away from office, 120
  printed instruction forms to pharmacist, 117–118
  reading time, 116
  routine procedures, 118
  rubber stamps, 118
  self-administered history forms, 118
  simple records, 117
  stair climbing, 117
  standard fee schedule, 118
  standing preadmission orders, 118
  telephone screening, 118
  traffic flow patterns, 118
Physicians' earnings ratio, 22
Pilling, Loran F., 65
Portability (*see* Pension plans)

Practice growth, effect of attitude on, 55–56
Practice management, 21
Practice management consultant, 32–34
  getting money's worth from, 32–33
Practice philosophy (*see* Income)
Professional Consulting Services, Inc., 14
Professional corporation (*see* Incorporated practice)
Professional Economics and Management Employee Performance Appraisal *(figure)*, 131
Professional relations (*see* Management: twelve strategic approaches)
Profit Sharing Plan (*see* Pension plans)
P's. the four of Medical Practice Management (*see* Management techniques)
Psycho-Cybernetics, 176

R

Red Cross, 27
Referrals (*see* Patient referrals)
Regan, Louis J. 63
Rieger, Scott C., 153
Rogan, Thomas, 122
Roos-Loos Group, 71–72

S

Salesmanship, 49
San Joaquin Foundation, 91
Saxton, Adam, 21
Sedgewick, Bill, 84
Self-employed retirement plans, 102–107
  checklist comparison, 106
  contributions and benefits, 103
    contribution formula, 105
    defined benefit plans, 103
    defined contribution plans, 103
    distributions, 105
    employee contributions, 104
    estate tax exemption, 105–107
    $5,000 death benefit exclusion, 107
    forfeitures, 105
    integration with social security, 104–105
    limitations, 103–104
    participation, 102
    trustees, 107
    vesting, 102–103

Self-employed retirement plans *(cont'd)*
    corporate retirement compared to Keogh, 102–107
    Keogh plan, 102–107
Separate Account balances *(see* Pension plans)
Service Bureau for Doctors, 151
Severa, Rudolph M., 159–160
Signer, Franklin, 174
S.M.A.-12 *(see* Management: twelve strategic approaches)
Social security benefits *(see* Pension plans)
Social security costs, 100
Society of Medical-Dental Management Consultants, 152
Solo practice *(see* Country doctor)
    advice for surviving, 81–82
    benefits of, 80
    disadvantages, 80–81
    reasons for enduring, 82–83
Stair climbing, 117
Stamford Credit Rating Bureau, 159
Standard fee schedule, 118
Standing preadmission orders, 118
Statement, personal *(see* Personal finances)
Strategic management approaches *(see* Management: twelve strategic approaches)
SUCCESS, acronym of Maxwell Maltz, 176
Suit-prone doctor *(see* Malpractice claims)
Suit-prone patient *(see* Malpractice claims)
Supporting personnel *(see* Personnel)
Systems and policies *(see* Management: twelve strategic approaches)

T

Taft, William Howard, 70
Tan, C. M., 47
Taxation exclusion *(see* Incorporated practice)
Tax savings *(see* Estate trusts)
Telephone patterns *(see* Patient: telephone patterns)

"Thank you," saying *(see* Management: twelve strategic approaches)
Thieman, E. A. "Bud," 151
Third party involvements *(see* Management: twelve strategic approaches)
Three-on-page checkbook *(see* Office procedures: practice income)
Tipping, James A., 152
Traisman, Howard, 171
Trusts, advice on *(see* Estate planning)

U

Unit Benefit Pension Plan *(see* Pension plans)

V

Van Horn, Dean, 139, 140
Vesting *(see* Pension plans)
Visiting Nurse Association, the, 27
Voltaire, 41

W

Wakelee, Albert T., 153
Walsh, Charles H., 34
Waste preventing actions *(see* Office staff)
White, Richard, 77–78
Will *(see* Estate planning)

Y

Young, David, 29–30

Z

Zolman, 66–67, 68